Success in Academic Surgery

Series editors
Lillian Kao
University of Texas Health Science Center at Houston
Houston, TX, USA

Herbert Chen
University of Alabama
Birmingham, AL, USA

T0276119

For further volumes:
http://www.springer.com/series/11216

Rachel R. Kelz • Sandra L. Wong

Editors

Surgical Quality Improvement

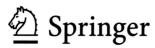 Springer

Editors
Rachel R. Kelz
University of Pennsylvania
Perelman School of Medicine
Philadelphia, PA
USA

Sandra L. Wong
The Geisel School of Medicine at
Dartmouth
Hanover, NH
USA

ISSN 2194-7481 ISSN 2194-749X (electronic)
Success in Academic Surgery
ISBN 978-3-319-23355-0 ISBN 978-3-319-23356-7 (eBook)
DOI 10.1007/978-3-319-23356-7

Library of Congress Control Number: 2016959034

This Springer imprint is published by Springer Nature
The registered company is Springer International Publishing AG
The registered company is Gewerbestrasse 11, 6330 Cham, Switzerland

Contents

Contributors

Peter Angelos MacLean Center for Clinical Medical Ethics, University of Chicago Med Center, Chicago, IL, USA

Megan K. Applewhite Department of Surgery and Alden March Bioethics Institute, Albany Medical College, Albany, NY, USA

Stanley W. Ashley Harvard Medical School, Boston, MA, USA

Brigham and Women's Hospital, Boston, MA, USA

Karl Y. Bilimoria Department of Surgery, Northwestern Memorial Hospital, Chicago, IL, USA

Justin B. Dimick Division of Minimally Invasive Surgery, Center for Healthcare Outcomes and Policy, Ann Arbor, MI, USA

Department of Surgery, University of Michigan, Ann Arbor, MI, USA

Scott Ellner General Surgery & Trauma Surgery, Saint Francis Hospital and Medical Center, Hartford, CT, USA

Bruce L. Hall Division of Research and Optimal Patient Care, American College of Surgeons, Department of Surgery, Washington University in St. Louis, St. Louis, MO, USA

Elliott R. Haut Division of Acute Care Surgery, Department of Surgery, The Johns Hopkins University School of Medicine, Baltimore, MD, USA

The Johns Hopkins University Bloomberg School of Public Health, Baltimore, MD, USA

Andrew M. Ibrahim Institute for Healthcare Policy & Innovation, University of Michigan, Ann Arbor, MI, USA

General Surgery, University Hospitals Case Medical Center, Ann Arbor, MI, USA

Kamal M. F. Itani Surgical Service, VA Boston Healthcare System, West Roxbury, MA, USA

Lillian S. Kao Division of Acute Care Surgery, Department of Surgery, University of Texas at Houston, Houston, TX, USA

Rachel R. Kelz Perelman School of Medicine, University of Pennsylvania, Piladelphia, PA, USA

Clifford Y. Ko Division of Research and Optimal Patient Care, American College of Surgeons, Department of Surgery, University of California Los Angeles, David Geffen School of Medicine, Veterans Affairs Greater Los Angeles Healthcare System, Los Angeles, CA, USA

Brandyn D. Lau Johns Hopkins University School of Medicine, Baltimore, MD, USA

Ira L. Leeds Department of Surgery, The Johns Hopkins Hospital, Baltimore, MD, USA

Jason B. Liu Clinical Scholar in Residence, American College of Surgeons, Chicago, IL, USA

Ryan D. Macht Department of Surgery, Boston University School of Medicine, Boston Medical Center, Boston, MA, USA

Martin A. Makary Johns Hopkins University School of Medicine, Health Policy & Management, Johns Hopkins Bloomberg School of Public Health, Baltimore, MD, USA

David McAneny Department of Surgery, Boston University School of Medicine, Boston Medical Center, Boston, MA, USA

Christina A. Minami Department of Surgery, Northwestern Memorial Hospital, Chicago, IL, USA

Brad S. Oriel VA Boston Healthcare System, Tufts University School of Medicine, Boston, MA, USA

Morgan M. Sellers Department of Surgery, Icahn School of Medicine at Mount Sinai, New York, NY, USA

Jo Shapiro Center for Professionalism and Peer Support, Department of Surgery, Brigham and Women's Hospital, Boston, MA, USA

Harvard Medical School, Boston, MA, USA

James Taylor General Surgery Resident, Department of Surgery, Johns Hopkins University School of Medicine, Baltimore, MD, USA

Lawrence C. Tsen Center for Professionalism and Peer Support, Department of Anesthesiology, Perioperative and Pain Medicine, Brigham and Women's Hospital, Boston, MA, USA

Harvard Medical School, Boston, MA, USA

Affan Umer General Surgery, UConn Health Center, Farmington, CT, USA

Elizabeth C. Wick Department of Surgery, University of California, San Francisco, CA, USA

Sandra L. Wong The Geisel School of Medicine at Dartmouth, Hanover, NH, USA

Tim Xu Department of Surgery, Johns Hopkins University School of Medicine, Baltimore, MD, USA

Anthony D. Yang Department of Surgery, Northwestern Memorial Hospital, Chicago, IL, USA

Chapter 1
Quality Improvement in Surgery

Lillian S. Kao

Abstract Surgeons can no longer afford to distance themselves from quality improvement (QI) initiatives given external pressures and disincentives from governing agencies as well as public demand for transparency and outcomes reporting. Multiple needs exist for conducting successful QI including higher quality and more sufficient evidence to guide care, better understanding of effective and context-sensitive implementation strategies, improved metrics with which to gauge successes and failures, and more resources and QI training for surgeons. Furthermore, surgeons face unique challenges in terms of assuming individual responsibility for outcomes that are a result of team-based care, measuring and adjusting for technical skill, and balancing technological and technical innovations with patient safety concerns. Despite these challenges, surgeons are leading the way in terms of the development of robust clinical registries with which to inform and drive QI, formation of local collaboratives to identify and drill down on variations in care and their impact on outcomes, and innovation in interventions to improve both individual and team-level outcomes such as video-based coaching and simulation-based training.

Introduction

Since the publication of the Institute of Medicine Report, "To Err is Human", significant strides have been made towards quality improvement (QI) in surgery. Several major QI initiatives such as those to reduce surgical infectious complications and to increase surgical safety checklist use have been driven by national organizations such as the Centers for Medicare and Medicaid Services, Joint Commission, and the World Health Organization. Other initiatives such as the development of robust clinical registries and of statewide collaboratives have been initiated by surgeons themselves. The success of these initiatives has been variable and often difficult to measure. Nonetheless, valuable lessons have been learned from these initiatives that can help guide the future of surgical QI.

L.S. Kao, MD, MS, CMQ
Division of Acute Care Surgery, Department of Surgery, University of Texas at Houston,
5656 Kelley Street, Houston, TX, 77026-1967, USA
e-mail: Lillian.S.Kao@uth.tmc.edu

© Springer International Publishing Switzerland 2017
R.R. Kelz, S.L. Wong (eds.), *Surgical Quality Improvement*,
Success in Academic Surgery, DOI 10.1007/978-3-319-23356-7_1

1

This chapter will provide a broad overview of the current needs in surgical QI. In particular, challenges specific to surgery will be described. Many of the topics mentioned in this chapter will be expanded on throughout the book.

Where Are We Now?

One of the first challenges encountered by the surgical community was the availability of robust, risk- and reliability-adjusted data upon which to base QI efforts. Currently, such data is primarily derived from one of two sources: (1) administrative databases which are comprised of claims data provided to health insurers and (2) clinical registries which are populated from review of patient charts. Both sources have their advantages and disadvantages. Administrative databases include Medicare and Medicaid databases, state hospital discharge datasets, Healthcare Cost and Utilization Project hospital databases, and the University Healthsystem Consortium database. They are readily available and relatively inexpensive to obtain, and they tend to include data on regional or well-defined populations. Outcomes such as mortality and length of stay are well-documented; however, accuracy of morbidity can be variable and highly dependent upon coding. Clinical registries use standardized definitions and trained abstractors to record data. Examples include the Society of Thoracic Surgeons National Database established in 1989 and the American College of Surgeons National Surgical Quality Improvement Project (ACS NSQIP) that started in 1991 as the National Veterans Administration Risk Study. Because participation in these clinical registries requires trained abstractors, this increases the costs, resources, and time necessary to obtain the data. However, the granularity of the data allows for more accurate assessment of morbidity and for robust risk adjustment. Multiple studies have compared administrative and data and identified significant differences between the two. Nonetheless, surgeons can use one or both sources of data to direct and evaluate surgical QI, as long as the limitations of each are understood.

Although data is necessary to drive surgical QI, it is not sufficient. This assertion is supported by two large database analyses published in the Journal of the American Medical Association (JAMA) in 2015 that demonstrated that participation in a surgical outcomes reporting program alone does not improve care (Etzioni et al. 2015; Osborne et al. 2015). Dr. Donald Berwick, former President and Chief Executive Officer of the Institute for Healthcare Improvement and prior Administrator of the Centers for Medicare and Medicaid services, cautioned however against interpreting these studies as a reason not to systematically measure and report outcomes (Berwick 2015). Rather, he emphasized the need for a process by which to learn from the data and to facilitate change locally. Similarly, Dr. Darrell Campbell Jr, the Program Director of the Michigan Surgical Quality Collaborative (MSQC), had stated in a perspective article several years earlier that "Quality Improvement is Local", meaning that there must be a mechanism by which providers interact locally to utilize the data in a meaningful manner to achieve improvements in patient care

(Campbell 2009). One mechanism by which surgeons have successfully translated data into improvements in outcomes is through collaboratives; examples include the MSQC and the Surgical Clinical Outcomes Assessment Program (SCOAP). Such collaboratives, whether they are regionally or procedurally based, build on robust data platforms and utilize strategies such as face-to-face sharing of evidence-based best practices to facilitate changes in surgical care.

The development of robust clinical registries and of successful collaboratives has greatly advanced surgical QI. Nonetheless, there are still significant strides to be made in optimizing the care of surgical patients. Several needs currently exist in order to further advance surgical QI.

Current Needs in Surgical QI

One pressing need is for the rapid yet rigorous generation of evidence for effective interventions to improve surgical outcomes. Generating data speedily and ensuring the external validity of the data are often viewed as opposing goals of clinical trials. Early adoption of promising interventions that have only been tested in a single-center randomized trial (or based on even less rigorous data) can result in significant harms if that intervention is subsequently proven to be ineffective or harmful (i.e., tight glycemic control with intensive insulin therapy). On the other hand, waiting for adequately-powered, high-quality, multi-center trials to demonstrate benefit may delay implementation of effective interventions. Furthermore, even when multiple randomized trials and meta-analyses have been performed, the effectiveness of various interventions remains controversial (i.e., mechanical bowel preparation to prevent surgical site infection after colon surgery). Strategies for addressing this challenge might include using alternative study designs such as the stepped wedge trial when the intervention is deemed to be low-risk. In a stepped wedge trial, the intervention is implemented at multiple sites in a random order such that each site serves as its own control and as a control for other sites. This design allows all sites to benefit from the intervention and is less susceptible to temporal trends. For example, this design was utilized in a multi-center trial evaluating the surgical safety checklist (Haugen et al. 2015). Another strategy is to use large observational datasets and advanced statistical methods such as instrumental variable analysis to make causal inferences. Additional strategies are necessary for rapidly generating large-scale data with minimal bias to identify effective interventions to improve surgical outcomes.

A second need is for strategies for effective and efficient implementation of evidence-based practices across multiple settings. Once an evidence-based practice has been proven effective, the challenge is in ensuring its uptake into routine practice across multiple settings. An example of an ongoing challenge is that of hand-washing; despite evidence of benefit, compliance with hand-washing remains a significant problem in many healthcare institutions. Dissemination and implementation science is an emerging field of inquiry for healthcare providers and researchers interested in minimizing the delays of putting research into practice. Dissemination refers to the distribution of information and materials about evidence-based interventions to targeted audiences, while implementation refers to the adoption of those interventions into routine practice in specific settings. Dissemination and implementation science provides theories and models upon which to base and evaluate interventions to increase the spread and uptake of evidence-based practices. The use of these theories allows researchers to compare results and improve the generalizability of their findings. However, this field is still evolving and challenges persist such as the lack of validation and harmonization of research measures used in these types of studies. Further discussion of the science of QI can be found in Chap. 2.

A third need is for appropriate measures upon which to assess the success or failure of surgical QI efforts. Traditional metrics include: (1) process measures such as the administration of appropriate spectrum antibiotics within an hour prior to incision, (2) outcome measures such as length of stay and mortality, and (3) patient-reported outcome measures such as health-related quality of life and patient satisfaction. There are advantages and disadvantages to each type of measure. For example, process measures provide actionable, real-time data that does not require advanced statistical techniques to analyze and that allows for targeted QI interventions. On the other hand, process measures may not be backed by high quality evidence or may too narrowly focus on one aspect of a quality problem. Furthermore, compliance with a process measure may not reflect fidelity, or performance of the intervention in the manner in which it was intended.

Improvements in one type of metric are not always associated with similar improvements in other types of metrics. For example, although process measures tend to be evidence-based, compliance with such process measures is not always associated with improved outcomes. In 2003, the Surgical Infection Prevention project was initiated with the goal of reducing postoperative surgical site infections by increasing use of appropriate perioperative antibiotic prophylaxis. Subsequently, the Surgical Care Improvement Project (SCIP) was developed by a partnership of ten national organizations to reduce postoperative infectious, cardiovascular, respiratory, and thromboembolic complications 25 % by 2010. Unfortunately, despite widespread endorsement of SCIP by greater than 30 organizations and despite increased adherence to the process measures, this program failed to result in the expected improvements in outcome (Ingraham et al. 2010; Stulberg et al. 2010). In another example, compliance with process measures and favorable surgical outcomes such as shorter lengths of stay have not been demonstrated to correlate to patient satisfaction (Kennedy et al. 2014). Measurement challenges in QI are addressed in more depth in Chap. 4.

A fourth need is for validated and standardized tools to measure context, which includes factors that contribute to the success of QI but do not include the methods or interventions themselves. Studies have demonstrated the importance of various aspects of context on the effectiveness of QI interventions. For example, the magnitude of reduction in morbidity with the surgical safety checklist has been correlated with changes in safety culture as measured by the Safety Attitudes Questionnaire (Haynes et al. 2011). Contextual factors important in QI include infrastructure, culture, and leadership at the local level. However, despite experts' ability to recognize those healthcare institutions with a context favorable towards good outcomes, no standardized tools are widely accepted for quantifying and evaluating context. For example, in a study of site visits to high and low outliers in ACS NSQIP for surgical site infections, all of the site visitors were able to identify whether hospitals were high or low outliers with 100 % accuracy (Campbell et al. 2008). Although the study was able to identify factors associated with high-performing hospitals, there was no composite measure that captured the site visitors' gestalt regarding context. The ideal tool would measure more than one aspect of context and would correlate contextual factors to patient outcomes and/or to success in QI. Furthermore, such a tool could be used to assess the effectiveness of interventions to improve context. For example, multiple interventions such as teamwork training have been demonstrated to improve specific aspects of context, namely related to safety culture (i.e., teamwork, communication, and safety climate) (Sacks et al. 2015). Lastly, accurate measurement of context may allow for development of more effective, context-sensitive implementation strategies of evidence-based practices. Chapter 6 will discuss the role of culture and communication in effective local surgical QI efforts.

A fifth need is for the training, personnel, and resources necessary to conduct surgical QI. Although the Accreditation Council for Graduate Medical Education (ACGME) has developed the Clinical Learning Environment Review (CLER) program to engage trainees in promoting safe and high quality patient care, there is a lack of evidence regarding the most effective strategies for educating trainees on QI. The Association of Program Directors in Surgery and the ACS NSQIP Quality In-Training Initiative are working to address this need through the development of materials and tools on quality improvement for use in surgical education. However, many currently practicing surgeons have not had any formal training in the tenets of QI and must rely on the available resources at their institutions that are often not specific to surgery. Participation in regional collaboratives, such as the Illinois Surgical Quality Improvement Collaborative (ISQIC, www.isqic.org) may provide institutions and surgeons with additional resources such as formal QI training, mentors, and process improvement consultants. Chapter 10 will further elucidate the current needs and principles in teaching QI.

Challenges Specific to Surgical QI

Surgical QI entails unique challenges. One particular challenge is that although optimizing surgical outcomes requires multi-disciplinary team-based care, individual surgeons are often held solely accountable for complications. Surgeons have traditionally been trained to accept responsibility for the team when adverse events occur; however, this adage has significant implications today. As the desire for transparency increases, so do the demands for public reporting of surgeon-specific surgical outcomes. For example, in 2015, ProPublica, an independent non-profit journalism group, released their Surgeon Scorecard which reported individual surgeons' outcomes on eight elective procedures based on 5 years' worth of Medicare data (https://projects.propublica.org/surgeons/). Although opponents of public reporting contend that surgical QI should be hospital-based (reflecting team efforts), ProPublica has argued that half of all US hospitals have both high and low performing surgeons. In addition, they propose that even after adjusting for patient and hospital factors, significant variation in surgeon performance exists. Surgeons' concerns regarding individual reporting include small sample sizes upon which the data are based, misinterpretation of the data by the public, and lack of validity of the outcome metrics (Sherman et al. 2013). Furthermore, consequences of such reports may lead to lack of acceptance of high-risk patients by many surgeons and misperceptions of surgeons' outcomes. Further work is necessary to ensure reporting of accurate and easily interpreted data that can be used to direct surgical QI.

A second challenge unique to surgical QI is the need to consider technical skills in interpreting surgical outcomes. Risk-adjustment strategies typically focus on patient-related factors with adjustment for hospital-level characteristics. However, these adjustments do not account for individual surgeons' technical skill. Data from a QI collaborative, the Michigan Bariatric Surgery Collaborative (MBSC), has demonstrated a relationship between technical skill of individual surgeons and postoperative outcomes in patients undergoing laparoscopic gastric bypass (Birkmeyer et al. 2013). Patients operated on by surgeons with low versus high skills as rated using a validated metric were at least twice as likely to die, have a complication, undergo reoperation, or be readmitted to the hospital. Thus, while public reporting of individual surgeon performance requires further refinement, that issue should not diminish the need to focus on individual surgeon performance to improve patient outcomes. Initiatives such as use of peer-to-peer video-based coaching are being studied currently in the MBSC as a potential mechanism for improving quality (Greenberg et al. 2016).

A third challenge is the tension between surgical innovation and patient safety. Surgeons continually encounter new technologies and/or techniques that have the potential to improve patient outcomes. However, the evidence for the safety and effectiveness of those innovations may be limited. Alternatively, the learning curve for effectively adopting those innovations may be unknown. In addition, there are ethical considerations regarding the need for human subjects approval and/or explicit informed consent for the innovation. The Society of University Surgeons issued a position statement recommending the formation of local Surgical Innovations Committees (SICs) and the use of a national registry for surgical innovations (Biffl et al. 2008). The position statement also provided indications for when surgical innovations require formal review. Development and adoption of formal guidelines that facilitate surgical innovation without compromising patient safety are necessary to ensure further advances in surgical care.

Conclusion

In conclusion, surgeons can no longer afford to distance themselves from QI initiatives given external pressures and disincentives from governing agencies as well as public demand for transparency and outcomes reporting. Multiple needs exist for conducting successful QI including higher quality and more sufficient evidence to guide care, better understanding of effective and context-sensitive implementation strategies, improved metrics with which to gauge successes and failures, and more resources and QI training for surgeons. Furthermore, surgeons face unique challenges in terms of assuming individual responsibility for outcomes that are a result of team-based care, measuring and adjusting for technical skill, and balancing technological and technical innovations with patient safety concerns. Despite these challenges, surgeons are leading the way in terms of the development of robust clinical registries with which to inform and drive QI, formation of local collaboratives to identify and drill down on variations in care and their impact on outcomes, and innovation in interventions to improve both individual and team-level outcomes such as video-based coaching and simulation-based training. This book will provide critical information on surgical QI to serve as a framework for thinking about these issues and a launching pad for improvement.

References

Berwick DM. Measuring surgical outcomes for improvement: was Codman wrong? JAMA. 2015;313(5):469–70.

Biffl WL, Spain DA, Reitsma AM, Minter RM, Upperman J, Wilson M, et al. Responsible development and application of surgical innovations: a position statement of the Society of University Surgeons. J Am Coll Surg. 2008;206(6):1204–9.

Birkmeyer JD, Finks JF, O'Reilly A, Oerline M, Carlin AM, Nunn AR, et al. Surgical skill and complication rates after bariatric surgery. N Engl J Med. 2013;369(15):1434–42.

Campbell Jr DA. Quality improvement is local. J Am Coll Surg. 2009;209(1):141–3.

Campbell Jr DA, Henderson WG, Englesbe MJ, Hall BL, O'Reilly M, Bratzler D, et al. Surgical site infection prevention: the importance of operative duration and blood transfusion--results of the first American College of Surgeons-National Surgical Quality Improvement Program Best Practices Initiative. J Am Coll Surg. 2008;207(6):810–20.

Etzioni DA, Wasif N, Dueck AC, Cima RR, Hohmann SF, Naessens JM, et al. Association of hospital participation in a surgical outcomes monitoring program with inpatient complications and mortality. JAMA. 2015;313(5):505–11.

Greenberg CC, Dombrowski J, Dimick JB. Video-based surgical coaching: an emerging approach to performance improvement. JAMA Surg. 2016;151(3):282–3.

Haugen AS, Softeland E, Almeland SK, Sevdalis N, Vonen B, Eide GE, et al. Effect of the World Health Organization checklist on patient outcomes: a stepped wedge cluster randomized controlled trial. Ann Surg. 2015;261(5):821–8.

Haynes AB, Weiser TG, Berry WR, Lipsitz SR, Breizat AH, Dellinger EP, et al. Changes in safety attitude and relationship to decreased postoperative morbidity and mortality following implementation of a checklist-based surgical safety intervention. BMJ Qual Saf. 2011;20(1):102–7.

Ingraham AM, Cohen ME, Bilimoria KY, Dimick JB, Richards KE, Raval MV, et al. Association of surgical care improvement project infection-related process measure compliance with risk-adjusted outcomes: implications for quality measurement. J Am Coll Surg. 2010;211(6):705–14.

Kennedy GD, Tevis SE, Kent KC. Is there a relationship between patient satisfaction and favorable outcomes? Ann Surg. 2014;260(4):592–8; discussion 8–600.

Osborne NH, Nicholas LH, Ryan AM, Thumma JR, Dimick JB. Association of hospital participation in a quality reporting program with surgical outcomes and expenditures for Medicare beneficiaries. JAMA. 2015;313(5):496–504.

Sacks GD, Shannon EM, Dawes AJ, Rollo JC, Nguyen DK, Russell MM, et al. Teamwork, communication and safety climate: a systematic review of interventions to improve surgical culture. BMJ Qual Saf. 2015;24(7):458–67.

Sherman KL, Gordon EJ, Mahvi DM, Chung J, Bentrem DJ, Holl JL, et al. Surgeons' perceptions of public reporting of hospital and individual surgeon quality. Med Care. 2013;51(12):1069–75.

Stulberg JJ, Delaney CP, Neuhauser DV, Aron DC, Fu P, Koroukian SM. Adherence to surgical care improvement project measures and the association with postoperative infections. JAMA. 2010;303(24):2479–85.

Chapter 2
The Science of Quality Improvement

Christina A. Minami, Karl Y. Bilimoria, and Anthony D. Yang

Abstract In order to carry out meaningful PI in healthcare, it is important to understand the main methodologies and their origins. The philosophies used in PI in healthcare originated in the mechanized world of industry. In this chapter, an overview of the PDSA (Plan-Do-Study-Act) cycle, Six Sigma, Lean, Lean Six Sigma, and the DMAIC (Define-Measure-Analyze-Improve-Control) frameworks will be provided, along with examples of published surgical QI projects that have made use of these methodologies. Though differences exist between these approaches, they all provide a step-wise, iterative approach to finding solutions to a defined and measurable problem.

Introduction

The most commonly used methodologies of surgical quality improvement (QI) are process improvement (PI) tools adopted from industry. W. Edwards Deming PhD, a physicist and leader in applied statistics, is credited for popularizing many of the modern PI philosophies. As one of the key figures in Japan's rise to an economic powerhouse in the latter half of the twentieth century, Deming became a hero abroad before his American colleagues recognized the profundity of his organizational philosophies (https://deming.org/). In the book, *Out of Crisis*, he outlined fourteen key principles in PI. The last point emphasized the need for engagement in the process, "Put everybody in the company to work to accomplish the transformation" (Kubiak and Benbow 2005).

This idea was echoed in 2012 by the Institute for Healthcare Improvement's CEO, who stated that everyone in health care should have two jobs: to do the work and to improve how the work is done (Scoville and Little 2014). This challenge has been accepted by the surgical world. Training current and future surgeons to undertake QI projects has become a major focus as governing bodies like the Accreditation Council for Graduate Medical Education (ACGME), the American Board of

C.A. Minami, MD (✉) • K.Y. Bilimoria, MD, MS • A.D. Yang, MD
Department of Surgery, Northwestern Memorial Hospital,
633 N St. Clair St 20th Floor, Chicago, IL 60611, USA
e-mail: ayang@nm.org

© Springer International Publishing Switzerland 2017
R.R. Kelz, S.L. Wong (eds.), *Surgical Quality Improvement*,
Success in Academic Surgery, DOI 10.1007/978-3-319-23356-7_2

Decrease in ABG Utilization Through Implementation of End Tidal CO2 Monitoring

Project Overview

Linkage to Strategic Plan: Provide the highest quality, most effective and safest care.

Problem Statement: Although a ventilation management protocol exists, awareness of the protocol and effective implementation of the Protocol in managing ventilation patients and weaning them from the ventilator is inconsistent. There is underutilization of ancillary tools to assess ventilator status and assist with ventilator weaning, specifically End- Tidal CO_2 monitors. Ineffective resource utilization results in increased reliance on arterial blood gas (ABG) measurements during ventilator weaning, a practice that has been shown to be unneccessary in the literature.

Goal/Benefit: Decrease the use of ABG measurements for mechanically ventilated patients in the surgical intensive care unit by implementation of routine End-Tidal CO_2 monitoring and emphasizing use of $ETCO_2$ & SpO_2 in place of arterial blood gas measurements, with the goal of reducing the overall cast of an ICU stay while still enabling effective ventillator weaning with no increase in ventilator duration.

Scope: Surgical Intensive Care Unit

System Capabilities/ Deliverables: Identification of current arterial blood gas utilization; implementation of surgical intensive care unit resident/nursing/respiratory therapy education on use of End-Tidal CO_2 monitoring in ventilator weaning anf appropriate ABG indications; implementation of end tidal CO_2 monitoring as a cost-effective alternative to arterial blood gas monitoring.

Resources Required: RT resource coordinators in SICU; RTs and RNs; IT for assistance with Powerchart documentation as well as EDW data mining for arterial blood gas utilization data and ventilator duration reports, RT to provide $EtCO_2$ monitors.

Key Metrics	Milestone		
Outcome Metric(s): • # of ABGs per patient-vent day • # of $ETCO_2$ recordings per patient-vent day **Process Metrics(s):** • % of patients with ETCO2 value recorded	**Description:** Approve Project Charter Identify baseline utilization rates Implement improvements Measure impact Establish control plan		**Date:** XXX, 20XX XXX, 20XX XXX, 20XX XXX, 20XX XXX, 20XX

Executive Sponsor:_____   Clinical Sponsor:_____   Sponsor:_____
Process Owner:_____   Improvement Leader:_____   Team Menbers:_____

D → M → A → I → C →

Fig. 2.1 Sample QI project charter

Medical Specialties (ABMS), and the Lucian Leape Institute at the National Patient Safety Foundation have called for formal education in patient safety and QI (Rhodes and Biester 2007).

In order to carry out meaningful PI in healthcare, it is important to understand the main methodologies and their origins. The philosophies used in PI in healthcare originated in the mechanized world of industry. In this chapter, an overview of the PDSA (Plan-Do-Study-Act) cycle, Six Sigma, Lean, Lean Six Sigma, and the DMAIC (Define-Measure-Analyze-Improve-Control) frameworks will be provided, along with examples of published surgical QI projects that have made use of these methodologies (Fig. 2.1). Though differences exist between these approaches, they all provide a step-wise, iterative approach to finding solutions to a defined and measurable problem.

PDSA

The Plan-Do-Study-Act Cycle (also known as the Deming Wheel or Deming Cycle) originated with Deming's mentor, Walter Shewhart (https://deming.org/). Deming, while working in Japan, eventually amended it to the Plan-Do-Check-Act (PDCA), but the basic principles stayed the same. This four-stage cycle is meant to structure continual improvement of a given process or product.

There are different frameworks that can be used to structure the approach to the PDSA cycle: both the MFI (Model For Improvement) and FOCUS frameworks have been well described. The MFI consists of three lead-in questions prior to entering the PDSA cycle: What are we trying to accomplish? How will we know if a change is an improvement? What change can we make that will results in an improvement? (Langley 2009) The FOCUS acronym refers to a more detailed pre-PDSA approach, requiring one to *Find* a process to improve, *Organize* a team that knows the process, *Clarify* current knowledge of the process, *Understand* causes of process variation, and *Select* the process improvement (Baltalden 1992).

Both MFI and FOCUS then lead to the PDSA cycle. In the Plan stage, objectives are set, a plan is defined, and a hypothesized outcome is articulated. In Do, the team implements the plan, documents any problems or unexpected findings, and begin their data analysis. In Study (or Check), data analysis is completed and the results are compared to the predicted outcomes. In Act, the team identifies further changes that need to be made and decides whether another PDSA cycle will be necessary (Administration HRaS 2011).

Part of the appeal of this approach to those working in healthcare improvement is PDSA's easy translation to the scientific method. Think of Plan as hypothesis formation, Do as the data collection period, Study as data analysis and interpretation, and Act as identifying problem areas that need to be addressed by future studies (Speroff and O'Connor 2004).

Examples of QI Projects in the Surgical Literature

The rise of QI/PI in surgery has led to the appearance of published QI projects in the literature. These publications can help to elucidate various approaches to common problems in surgery and facilitate the diffusion of rigorous QI/PI methods throughout the surgical community. In this chapter, we provide examples of different published projects that focus on a common problem in the surgical world: operating room (OR) efficiency. Though each of the projects feature a different methodological approach and implemented different interventions, they were all able to achieve their project aim.

Torkki et al's project (2006) used the PDCA cycle to address OR waiting times for trauma patients. In the Plan stage, the team defined what data was to be collected, including waiting time before surgery and time between operations. It was then decided that three areas would be targeted in the Do phase: anesthesia induction (instead of waiting for the preceding case to finish, induction was moved to pre-op areas), process guidance (a nurse coordinator was given the task of coordinating patient and OR personnel and calling for the next patient, and ORs were assigned by anticipated length of operation), and patient flow (trauma patients were relocated to the unit located closest to the ORs). In the Check stage, the team found that by implementing these changes, the average OR waiting time decreased by 20.5 % (p<0.05) and time between operations decreased by 23.1 % (p<0.001). Finally, in reflecting on the lessons learn in the Act stage, the team observed that although using process metrics (i.e. measuring steps in a given process) was helpful in understanding the entire flow of the patient in and out of the OR, they did identify the need to understand the effects on patient outcomes that may result from their process changes.

Six Sigma

Six Sigma was originally conceptualized by Motorola in the mid 1980s and is fundamentally a data-driven philosophy of improvement that values the prevention of defects over the detection of defects (Kubiak and Benbow 2005). Motorola declared that it would achieve a defect rate of no more than 3.4 parts per million within 5 years, which was to supposedly correlate to failure rates outside of six standard deviations (sigma) from the mean. Though some scholars have pointed out that this may not be strictly accurate (Pyzdek 1999), the moniker persist in the literature and, for all practical purposes, refers to a process quality goal of achieving as close to zero defects as possible (Kumar 2006). Xerox, General Electric, and Kodak soon followed Motorola's lead. All of these industrial giants identified their driving objective to create products and services that were nearly perfect by eliminating variation. In order to address this, the product life cycle had to be understood as a structured, customer-centric process, that generated a reliable, high-quality product at the lowest cost possible (Kumar 2006). Translating this to healthcare requires us to replace customers with patients or providers, products with healthcare services, and shareholders with all stakeholders in the healthcare industry (e.g. family members, caregivers, physicians, hospitals, payers, etc).

Inherent to the Six Sigma approach is the understanding that improvements happen over months to years, not days to weeks. In addition, implementation of Six Sigma is a team process, requiring engagement from the entire organization from the bottom to the top of the hierarchy. While front-line providers may be the ones carrying out the processes and improvements in question, executive leadership and senior management buy-in are indispensable to the organization's success in the Six Sigma philosophy.

Two main frameworks exist to practically address the improvement process of Six Sigma: DMADC (Define-Measure-Analyze-Design-Verify) and DMAIC. While DMADC focuses on the design of a product and is a prospective, proactive process, DMAIC looks at existing processes to fix problems and is usually characterized as a reactive process. DMAIC fits the improvement processes in healthcare much more readily and is thus described in detail here.

DMAIC acts as a roadmap that offers a clear organizational structure to the conceptualization of QI/PI projects. It can be applied to multiple clinical settings to improve processes and eliminate errors in complex environments. Each phase of DMAIC (Define, Measure, Analyze, Implement, Control) act as project milestones and can be complex undertakings in and of themselves. It should be emphasized that the entire PI process and each DMAIC phase represent *iterative* processes and QI teams should be ready to continually address the effects of process changes before undertaking a project.

Define

In the Define stage, the project's aim should be clearly articulated. This usually begins with a general sense of an inefficient or faulty process or with consistently poor clinical outcomes that need to be addressed. The main questions to be considered at this stage are, "What is the problem or improvement opportunity? Who does the problem affect and what are their expectations?"

Initial organization of the project centers around the project charter, which is the document that outlines the project's problem, specific quantitative goals, scope, required resources, key metrics, and team members. In general, a QI/PI project should address an important operational or clinical issue, have clear objectives that can are responsive to the needs of the "customers" (most often, patients), be tied back to the organization's overarching goal, have a committed sponsor and process owner(s), have readily-available data for measurement and ongoing performance evaluation, have an unknown solution, and be focused enough to be completed in 6–9 months.

Building an effective QI team is of high importance to the success of any QI project, and a good project team requires members from all levels of the organization's hierarchy. The *process owner* is the individual who is instrumental in the implementation of the project and who measures the project outputs and improvements. He/she works hand in hand with the *improvement leader*, who is usually a methodology expert and who ensures that the DMAIC framework is being properly applied to complete deliverables. The *executive sponsor* provides strategic oversight and address project barriers from the organizational level. *Sponsors*, can address lower-level barriers at the departmental level, and take responsibility for the timely and successful implementation of the project. The *clinical sponsor*, usually an attending-level physician who is knowledgeable and experienced in the clinical area that the project is addressing, helps to mediate decisions involving the clinical aspects of the project. Finally, the *team members* can be from a variety of different backgrounds, but all contribute to project ideas, data collection, data analytics, and project implementation (Schumacher 2012).

Tools that can be used in this phase include SIPOC diagrams, process flowcharts, and stakeholder analyses. SIPOC charts can give a high level overview of the process of interest and help to identify the customers involved with each step of the process. Each part of the acronym (Suppliers/Inputs/Process/Outputs/Customers) has its own column in the chart, and team members work to fill in each row sequentially. For instance, if a project is looking at flows in an emergency room, one of the Suppliers can be a physician, the Input would be a sick patient, Processes can include admission orders, Outputs include completed admission orders, and the customer would be a Nurse (Floriani 2010). This broad overview of the process may then naturally lead into more detailed mapping in the form of process flowcharts or targeted evaluations in the form of stake-holder analyses. Process flowcharts are graphic illustrations of processes that capture the flow and inter-relationships of the actions that lead to a product. Different shapes denote particular parts of the process (e.g., an oval shows the first or last step in a process, a rectangle depicts a particular task, an arrow shows the direction of the flow, and a dia-mond indicates a decision point) (HRSA 2015). Stakeholder analyses are less rigid in method, being straightforward evaluations of what the stakeholders need or expect from an organization. A guide to carrying out these evaluations may look like this: (1) identify the organization's stakeholders through a brainstorming session with team members, (2) classify the stakeholders into defined groups, (3) identify the needs and expectations of each group of stakeholders, and (4) using the insight generated by these conversations, develop strategies for addressing these needs and expectations (Andersen 2007). Process mapping and stakeholder analysis can provide a framework to begin thinking about failure points in the process of interest that can be improved.

Measure

In the Measure stage, the key metrics of the project have been identified and *baseline data* are gathered and analyzed in order to give the team a clear idea of their starting point. The two types of measures most commonly used in DMAIC projects are pro-cess measures, which are measures taken at defined points in a process of care and reflect values of the individual steps, and outcome measures. Thus, while both process and outcome measures can be indicative of the performance of the entire process (Kassardjian et al. 2015), both have their respective pros and cons. While outcomes measures are usually valid and stable (e.g. mortality and morbidity rates), and they reflect what patients usually care about, robust risk adjustment is required in order for any comparison to be valid and useful for QI. Outcomes are also the product of a complex, multifactorial process and thus do not necessarily help to measure particular aspects of the process in question. In addition, they are often plagued by low-event rates and long-horizon times (Donabedian 1966). As a result, it is often difficult to change outcomes in a short timeframe, sometimes limiting the practicality of outcome measures for use in a 6–9 month DMAIC project. Process measures may be more helpful in a QI/PI project, as data collection can be done while the process is occur-ring, and they do not require the use of risk adjustment. In addition, process measures can often be abstracted from data that are already recorded for clinical or administra-tive use and may not require additional collection of data elements as outcomes mea-sure might (Rubin et al. 2001). Particular attention does need to be paid to the specifications used to deem patient populations eligible for process measures, how-ever, and it can be difficult to summarize a process as a whole using data from mea-sures that are indicative of fragmentary parts (Rubin et al. 2001).

After the key metrics for a QI/PI project have been chosen, the team must then build a data collection plan and decide how to collect the data. Part of this plan must include delineating the *operational definition*, or a precise description of how to put a value to the measurable characteristic in question. For instance, if the team is

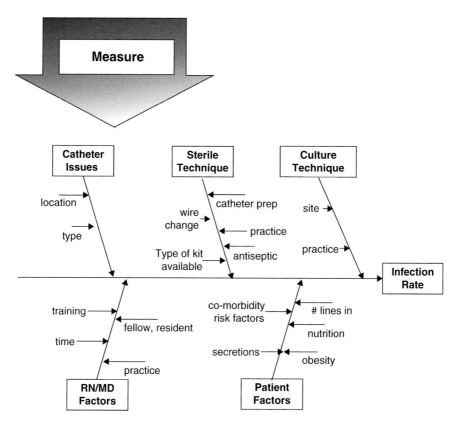

Fig. 2.2 Fishbone diagram of possible factors contributing to CR-BS. (Reproduced with permission from Frankel et al. (2005)

working on a project on reducing 30-day readmission in patients undergoing gastrointestinal surgery, how should the numerator and denominator be defined to obtain the readmission rate that is relevant to their QI goal? The operational definition of the readmission rate in this case can be calculated by dividing the number of inpatient readmissions to any hospital within 30-days of the index surgery by all patients undergoing gastrointestinal surgery (ISQIC (ISQIC) 2014).

Defining or choosing process metrics may be more difficult than with outcomes metrics. Using the Five Why's philosophy (iteratively asking "Why" multiple times until the true underlying driver of variation is identified) in light of a particular project's aims will allow for progressively more detailed answers as to what is driving variation in a process, and may help to identify key process metrics. Furthermore, identifying stratifications (e.g. figuring out the Who, What, When, and Where of a process) and detailed process maps are tools that can aid in identifying process metrics. A fishbone (or Ishikawa) diagram, which pictorially describes cause-and-effects in a process, in another way of drilling down to the drivers of process variation. The bones of the fish are the drivers of the process. A practical example is illustrated in Fig. 2.2, from a project focused on decreasing catheter-related bloodstream infections (CR-BSI) (Frankel et al. 2005).

Analyze

In the Analyze phase, the team should be able to *identify sources of variation*, and apply statistical tools to *identify key drivers of error and process variation*. Data analysis is important to this step, and this will lead to the generation of hypotheses as well as the verification and elimination of root causes. After baseline measurements are generated in the Measure phase and the process in question has been mapped, the team can leverage knowledge of the process and benchmark its baseline performance to validate their goal (Kassardjian et al. 2015).

In confirming their goal, teams should be careful to ensure that the project goals utilize the key metric(s) that was identified in the Measure phase. In addition, the goal can be validated by looking inward at an organization's best historical performance as well as looking outward, by using benchmarked measures to compare the organization's performance against an outside peer group. Goal validation also requires the team to be specific with regards to the type of change that is desired in their key metric. That is, is the goal to shift the mean of the organization's performance, reduce the variation, or both?

The identification of potential sources of variation started in the Measure stage; in Analyze, the number of candidate sources of variation for intervention should be narrowed. While all causes of error are important to keep in mind, the root causes represent the biggest targets for intervention as they are responsible for the majority of the variation. Root cause identification is performed through an iterative cycle of (1) exploring, (2) generating hypotheses regarding root causes, and (3) verifying or eliminating root causes (ISQIC 2014). There are several tools that QI teams can use to turn the data that they gather into useful, relevant information to guide their project. Examples of tools to *explore* the data collected include: Pareto charts (a bar graph that summarizes the relative importance of different groups or categories) (ASQ 2015), run charts (line graph depicting data over time), histograms (graphical representation of the shape of data distribution), and scatter diagrams (usually depicted with process measures as the independent variable and outcomes as the dependent variable). Stratifications, the Five Whys, process mapping, and fishbone diagrams can be added to help *generate hypotheses*. Control vs Impact tables (i.e., determining if drivers are in the team's control or not in their control, and assigning a level of impact of the intervention), and Failure Modes Effect Analysis (FMEA) can be used to *verify or eliminate causes*. An FMEA is an organized, systematic way to identify and analyze possible failure points in a process and to identify the relative importance of each "failure mode" through calculation of a risk priority number (RPN). Figure 2.3 is a template of an FMEA that can be carried out by hospital teams when addressing postoperative venous thromboembolism (VTE).

Improve

In the Improve stage, *solutions* ("*interventions*") to the problems identified and quantified in the preceding stages are selected and implemented. Creative solutions are generated through team brainstorming sessions. Participation is invited from all

Step 1: Identify Failure Modes and calculate a Risk Priority Number(RPN)
At your table, identify 3-5 potential failure points based on the high level VTE prophylaxis process. For each failure mode, assign a risk score of 1, 2 or 3 points for severity, frequency of occurrence, and probability that the failure would be detected and corrected before harm could occur. Refer to the key below for guidance.

Key	1	2	3
Severity: How bad is the effect?	Unlikely to increase risk of VTE	May increase risk of VTE	Likely to increase risk of VTE
Occurrence: How often does it happen?	< 20% of patients	20-40% of patients	> 40% of patients
Detection: When it happens do we know When do we know?	Immediate and automated	Recognized with effort	Undetectable until harm occurs or with significant effort

Calculate the Risk Priority Number (RPN) for each failure. RPN= Severity x Occurrence x Detection

Potential Failure Modes	Risk Score(1-3)			
	Severity	Occurrence	Detection	RPN
1				
2				
3				
4				
5				

Step 2: Prioritize Failure Modes and Identify Actions to Reduce Risk
The RPN helps you prioritize the top 2-3 potential failure modes. For each potential failure mode, identify specific actions that can be taken to reduce risk and improve performance of the VTE prophylaxis process.

Failure Modes 1:
Failure Modes 2:
Failure Modes 3:

Fig. 2.3 Template used in an FMEA exercise addressing processes affecting postoperative VTE

attendees, every idea proposed is documented, and the team must be careful to avoid shooting down the idea prematurely. Open brainstorming sessions, in which ideas are spontaneously called out, can be effective and there are ways of structuring the sessions. Structured idea-generating meeting strategies include: (1) a round-robin approach, in which team members call out solutions in turn, (2) the slip method, in which team members write all of their ideas down on paper and then pool and organize them, and (3) gallery walk, in which topics are set up around the room, and mini-brainstorming sessions are held at each topic area (ISQIC 2014). As potential solutions come under consideration, the process leader may guide the team by counseling them on some general improvement principles that can improve the chances of implementing a successful intervention. The team should look for solutions that reduce reliance on memory, are easy to carry out, use fail-safe systems, reduce handoffs, develop clear lines of accountability, and avoid reliance on a single individual. While a solution may not be able to fulfill all of these criteria, these principles can guide the prioritization of different ideas.

Teams can also generate a detailed process map that has not only current processes, but the anticipated new processes; including these possible future changes can help to identify any new and/or unanticipated downstream problems or risks that the proposed changes may introduce. At this stage, involvement of front-line staff is of primary importance as their expertise in clinical processes can be invaluable. In projects that involve streamlining processes, the following approaches often have a greater chance of being successful: simplifying the process, eliminating unnecessary handoffs, using parallel processes, creating alternative paths, or shifting resources to eliminate bottlenecks (ISQIC 2014).

The search for creative solutions may require one to look outside one's own organization. With the rise of state surgical quality improvement collaboratives (e.g. Washington state's Surgical Clinical Outcomes Assessment Program, Michigan's Surgical Quality Collaborative, Tennessee's Surgical Quality Collaborative, and Illinois' Surgical Quality Improvement Collaborative), comes the opportunity for hospitals to network with each other and learn what interventions worked or failed at everyone's respective institutions. In addition, interventions from outside the healthcare industry can be used successfully in healthcare QI, if they are adapted and translated effectively. One of the most well-known examples is the surgical checklist, which originated in the aviation industry (Gawande 2009). It grew into a global initiative that, in some studies, resulted in impressive improvements in patient outcomes (Haynes et al. 2009).

Once a particular solution has been chosen, obtaining buy-in from everyone involved in the change from the top of the hierarchy to front-line providers is essential to the success of the intervention. This is one of the most important parts of enacting change, and can be one of the most challenging. Gaining buy-in requires team members to think carefully about how to identify which aspects of their QI project will resonate with different levels of the institution. For instance, the hospital leadership may respond more positively to the publicly-reported performance improvements and financial benefits of the project, while front-line providers may respond better to how the project benefits patients or makes their job easier. Presentations to key stakeholders should be well-practiced and efficient, with clear graphics and visuals, a clear depiction of both the potential benefits and the potential costs, and allow for input from the audience.

Actual *implementation* of a change is a science in and of itself. Briefly, there are three different ways to approach implementing an intervention. First, teams may choose to implement easy, reversible, measurable parts of the intervention early in the process to generate "early wins," which can generate excitement amongst key stakeholders and facilitate further buy-in. Second, a pilot intervention may be used when change will be costly, difficult to reverse, and may result in unintended consequences. Third, in some cases, because of cost, time constraints, or technical requirements, the full scale intervention must "go-live" at once. This requires immaculate planning to anticipate any problems or unintended consequences and robust communication to ensure that all staff are aware of the change (ISQIC 2014).

Table 2.1 Strengths and weaknesses of various control mechanisms (Schumacher 2012; ISQIC 2015)

Effectiveness	Control mechanism	Strengths and weaknesses
Strong	Mistake Proofing	*Strengths*: can achieve a 0 % error rate; does not require training or feedback mechanisms *Weaknesses*: difficult to create and implement; can lead to a false sense of security
	Statistical Process Control	*Strengths*: enables identification of variation and changes; minimizes unnecessary use of resources *Weaknesses*: requires disciplined and complex measurement; difficult to interpret; requires timely feedback and corrective action; does not prevent errors
	Monitoring	*Strengths*: assists with accountability; provides feedback to leadership; provides data for problem solving *Weaknesses*: requires timely/structured review of results; requires corrective action ownership, does not prevent errors
	Standard Operating Procedures	*Strengths*: provides consistency via a standard process, assigns defined responsibilities *Weaknesses*: requires ownership/maintenance; only succeeds with training, requires monitoring for compliance, does not prevent errors
	Checklists	*Strengths*: serves as standard reference, can be used as a record, low cost *Weaknesses*: requires individual use and compliance, does not prevent errors
	Vigilance	*Strengths*: inspires personal ownership, engages staff, low cost *Weaknesses*: requires individual accountability, must be bolstered by successful communication, prone to fatigue, does not prevent errors
	Training	*Strengths*: engages staff, exposes staff to proper process *Weaknesses*: high cost, requires continued assessment, does not prevent errors from occurring
Weak	Communication	*Strengths*: engages staff, creates awareness, low cost *Weaknesses*: multiple layers of communication required, does not prevent errors

Control

Once the change has been implemented successfully, a control mechanism must be put in place to ensure ongoing consistent performance improvement. In this way, any positive changes resulting from a QI project will be sustained over the long-term. There is a sliding scale of effectiveness of standard control mechanisms (Table 2.1). Mechanisms known to be weak include: communication, training, and vigilance. Checklists, standard procedures, monitoring ("audit and feedback"), and statistical process control (which consists of measures taken over time with identification of extreme variation), are stronger structures, but are not error-proof (Schumacher 2012). True mistake-proofing occurs when defects are actually designed out of the process (e.g. forcing functions built into the electronic ordering system of a healthcare facility). In practice, however, true mistake-proofing is difficult to create and so it is the minority of interventions that can rely on a true error-proofed process.

Another key component of the Control phase is the continual tracking and monitoring of the key metrics. It is the process owner's responsibility to continue this monitoring, but the team needs to aid in creating an overall control plan. Ideally, automated data collection can be taken advantage of and a long-term plan for educating new staff members and/or refreshing existing staff's training should be put into place. When there is a sustained, negative change in performance (defined by the team in the creation of the control plan), there will be a mechanism in place to gather the team back together to examine the data, identify the cause of the drop in performance, and implement a targeted intervention to address the problem or failure identified by the team. In this way, improvements made over the course of the DMAIC process can be sustained.

One of the earliest instances of a published surgical Six Sigma project was by Adams and colleagues; their project aimed to improve general surgery OR turnaround time in order to decrease wasted time and financial costs (Adams et al. 2004). This project was initiated after the president of the healthcare system introduced Six Sigma and made it clear that the entire system would have to undergo PI training. It is important to note that this was a strong "top-down" approach, as the importance of Six Sigma was passed down from the president to the executive group, then to the hospital and system board, to the medical board, and then down to the physicians and hospital staff.

After all executives and staff underwent Six Sigma training, a multidisciplinary team was formed. Case turnaround times were abstracted from a 2 month period and mean baseline turnaround time was measured at 60.9 minutes with a standard deviation of 23.8 min. The turnaround process was broken down into three components: (1) surgeon-out to patient-out, (2) patient-out to patient-in, and (3) patient-in to surgeon-in. It was determined that different "waves" of the project would focus on different segments of the process. Further investigation demonstrated that more than 50 % of the variation in turnaround time arose from the patient-out to patient-in segment and so the specific aim of the first wave focused on decreasing this particular segment by a statistically significant amount. After process mapping and brainstorming, the team identified six improvement actions, including: (1) concurrent room cleanup and containment by the team, (2) cleanup and breakdown of the surgical setup immediately following wound closure and dressing application, (3) consistent staff assignments, (4) complete case carts, (5) consistent and timely notification of the surgeon of room readiness, and (6) increased assistance from anesthesia personnel. A Failure Modes and Effects Analysis (FMEA) was performed prior to implementation in order to identify potential downstream effects. Rollout of the initiative took place through multiple meetings with the OR staff and physician staff. Post-intervention results demonstrated that the patient-out to patient-in time decreased from 22.8 min to 15.6 min (z score = 2.13). The potential financial gains were estimated at $162,000 per year from potential additional OR cases. The team credited a handful of factors for their success: the initiative was leadership-driven, the team remained customer focused, the process was based on solid data, the staff were well trained in Six-Sigma methodology, and the organization had a strong desire to improve outcomes (Adams et al. 2004).

Lean

Lean manufacturing, often referred to simply as Lean, was first developed by Toyota Production Systems in the 1950s. Its applicability to healthcare arises from the fact that it is not merely a manufacturing tactic but is primarily a management strategy (Going Lean in Health Care 2005). As its name might suggest, this method is primarily concerned with waste (*muda*), or processes that do not add value to a product. Waste can take place in seven different areas: transportation, inventory, motion, waiting, overproduction, over-processing, and defects (Waring and Bishop 2010). Cutting this waste can be accomplished by applying the five principles of Lean thinking:

1. *Value* of a certain product is evaluated from the viewpoint of a customer's need. Within healthcare, value has three different dimensions: clinical value, or the achievement of the best possible patient outcome; operational value, referring to the efficiency, accessibility, and continuity of care; and experiential value, or the satisfaction of patients and healthcare workers alike (Goodridge et al. 2015).
2. The *value stream* refers to the production process, originating from the customer's need and extending through production to the point of consumption (Scoville and Little 2014). This encompasses the entire set of activities across all parts of the organization.
3. *Flow* should be present as the product progresses through the steps of the process. Waste should be eliminated and the service/product should be presented to the customer without detours, interruptions, or waiting.
4. Where flow is not possible, the principle of *pull*, should be present. This is the idea that the process is created around the organization's understanding of the customer's needs, producing not only *what* is desired but *when* it is desired (Goodridge et al. 2015).
5. *Perfection* is the theoretical endpoint, at which every part of the process adds value for the customer. *Kaizen*, or continual small improvements, is an overarching principle that can be applied to achieve this.

Waste in healthcare can come in different forms (Campbell 2009). Information waste (e.g. multiple intake forms that gather the same information or different data systems that cannot crosstalk with one another) is an example that many patients are probably familiar with. Physical environment waste is often seen in the OR, when

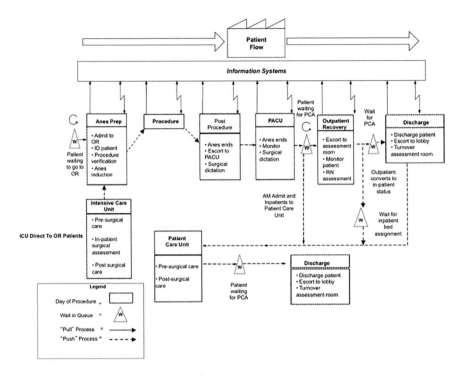

Fig. 2.4 Example of value-stream mapping of OR processes (Reproduced with permission from Cima et al. (2011))

supplies are opened and left unused. Process waste includes repeating tasks that have already been performed (e.g. redrawing a blood sample that was previously drawn but lost by the lab), time waste, and actual process defects resulting in patient harm or death.

As with the Six Sigma approach and the implementation of any DMAIC project, strong leadership is critical to the success of Lean. Some experts estimate that implementing Lean tools represent only about 20 % of the effort in Lean transformations, with the remaining 80 % spent on shifting leadership practices and behaviors (Mann 2009). Though this specific breakdown is debatable, the importance of Lean leaders is undeniable. They are supposed to operate as coaches and mentors, rather than adopting more distant roles as administrators. An all-inclusive culture, in which any staff member is invited to participate, as well as a no-blame approach to mistakes and errors is also part of the Lean approach (Goodridge et al. 2015).

Lean tools are similar to those detailed in the DMAIC section of this chapter, including process mapping, work and process observation, standardizing processes, use of checklists, and error proofing. Value-stream mapping is a technique that is more specific to Lean management. In these maps, processes are mapped along with information and material flows. By mapping current states, value-added and non-value-added steps can be identified and properly addressed (Fig. 2.4).

Also strongly associated with Lean are the concepts of *heijunka* and *kanban*. *Heijunka*, or process smoothing, is a method used by TPS to ensure that production meets demand in the relevant timeframe. A *heijunka* chart can be made with product types comprising the rows, and time units comprising the columns, thus allowing for a visual depiction of demand for different product types over time (http://leaninstituut.nl/publications/1106/The_Heijunka_Box.pdf). *Kanban* is a visual signaling system used to notify workers when new supplies are needed and in what quantity. It is used in materials management, in hospital storerooms and equipment areas. One example is taping a yellow square and a red square side-by-side in a storeroom; empty oxygen tanks can be placed in the red squares and full tanks placed in the yellow, allowed for employees to surmise the floor's supplemental oxygen supply at a quick glance (Zidel 2006).

An example of a successful Lean project that focused on OR efficiency used value-stream mapping (VSM) to decrease throughput time per patient (time into the OR to time out of the OR) (Schwarz et al. 2011). Their VSM detailed the processes of patient throughput, breaking it down into four components (waiting, transporting, running, and servicing). This map was used to identify process waste like time, human resources, and materials waste. In their particular institution, weak points and waste were identified in a number of different steps (e.g. waiting for the patient, waiting for the operating surgeon, short-notice changes to the OR plan, interdisciplinary communication problems). One of the mainstays of their intervention was changing the system from a Push (in which patients were transferred to the OR regardless of capacity) to a Pull system; that is, the patients were only transferred after the OR gave the go-ahead. The pre-op holding area was optimized to allow for anesthesia procedures that were originally carried out in the OR. Processes were performed in parallel whenever possible, such as closing one patient while disinfecting instruments, and calling for and preoperatively evaluating the following patient at the same time. After the intervention phase, the team was able to decrease the mean throughput time from 151 min to 120 min. Throughput has been continually monitored on an OR dashboard, allowing for direct feedback to OR personnel.

Lean Six Sigma

The synthesis of Lean and Six Sigma seem natural given that Lean guides overall organizational attitude and thinking and Six Sigma stresses an analytic framework for problem solving (Knapp 2015). Michael George, in his 2002 book, is credited for the creation of Lean Six Sigma. He pointed out that Six Sigma does not directly address the speed of processes and that companies that use only Six Sigma usually don't achieve improvement in lead time. On the other hand, George pointed out that when Lean methods are used alone, improvement is usually seen in small parts of companies rather than across whole corporations. He thus proposed Lean Six Sigma, which is "a methodology that maximizes shareholder value by achieving the fastest rate of improvement in customer satisfaction, cost, quality, process speed, and invested capital" (George 2002).

The combination leads to a system that boasts the Six Sigma organizational principles, embraces the philosophies of Lean, and combines their respective toolkits to allow organizations to "[do] quality quickly" (George 2002). Projects can either have a Lean-focused approach, which apply best practices and focus on implementing standard solutions to increase speed and reduce lead and processes time, or a Six Sigma-focused approach, which is often used in more complex problems that involve data-based analytic methods and stress control mechanisms. The DMAIC framework can be used in either case. In Lean Six Sigma, like both of its parents, organizational competency is a must, requiring dedicated training of project leaders and staff in PI methodology (de Koning et al. 2006).

Cima et al. (2011) applied these methodologies in their own project focused on increasing OR efficiency. The authors used the DMAIC framework and made robust use of statistical analysis and process metric collection to reduce process variation, while also using value-stream mapping to identify the value-added and non-value-added steps. They measured pre-intervention measures across three surgical specialties (thoracic, gynecologic, and general surgery), looking at on-time starts, operations running past 5 PM, turnover time, staff overtime, and change in operating margin. The project had a multidisciplinary leadership team and then used smaller teams to redesign five specific work streams: unplanned surgical volume variation, streamlining preoperative processes, reducing OR non-operative time, reducing redundancy of patient information collection, and employee engagement. Examples of process interventions carried out by the team included: streamlining preoperative processes by standardizing preoperative assessment criteria across all groups performing preoperative patient clearance; staggering OR start-times to promote on-time starts; and implementing parallel processing and preoperative procedure rooms to reduce OR non-operative time. After implementation of these changes, the QI team found that they were able to improve on-time OR starts, decrease the number of cases that ran past 5 PM, decrease turnover time, and decrease staff overtime. This improved efficiency led to improved OR financial performance, increasing operating margins by 16–51 %. This improvement was continued and also spread beyond the three surgical specialties studied, illustrating this project as a successful application of Lean Six Sigma to surgical quality improvement (Cima et al. 2011).

Conclusion

This chapter outlined some of the theoretical and practical basics of commonly used QI methodologies in healthcare. It should be noted, however, that effective QI learning requires more than the provision of reading materials; interactive training and practical, hands-on training in a supported setting is paramount. This type of training can be effective when housed within a single hospital, but can also be efficiently disseminated in training targeting larger multi-institutional organizations or even in large collaborative networks. For instance, the Illinois Surgical Quality Improvement

Collaborative (ISQIC), a statewide collaborative focused on disseminating QI teaching throughout its 55 participating hospitals is helping its member hospitals to achieve rapid, effective, and sustained quality improvement. ISQIC has prioritized equipping hospital surgical QI teams with the tools to implement data-driven QI through multiple modalities. PI methodology (DMAIC is used as the example) and QI principles have been taught to all surgical QI teams using customized online modules and in-person practice exercises (e.g., walking through a DMAIC project simulation and FMEA) at semi-annual collaborative meetings. Mentored implementation of QI through intensive support from an expert PI coach and the ISQIC coordinating center is also provided to hospitals in the collaborative.

Although the methodologies discussed here have different theoretical underpinnings and stress different aspects of process improvement, they all represent a stepwise, iterative approach to achieving higher quality. As our main examples illustrate, successful surgical QI in similar arenas can be carried out using PDSA, Six Sigma, Lean, or Lean Six Sigma. No matter what methodology underlies a given project, strong leadership, a supportive organizational culture, strong PI training, and a dedicated multidisciplinary team are essential to carrying out meaningful surgical QI. Surgeons should be encouraged to become experts in PI/QI methodology as surgeon leadership in QI is essential to achieve meaningful gains in the quality of patient care.

References

Adams R, Warner P, Hubbard B, Goulding T. Decreasing turnaround time between general surgery cases: a six sigma initiative. J Nurs Adm. 2004;34(3):140–8.

Administration HRaS. Testing for improvement 2011 [December 12, 2015]. Available from: http://www.hrsa.gov/quality/toolbox/methodology/testingforimprovement/part2.html.

Andersen B. Business process improvement toolbox. Milwaukee: ASQ Quality Press; 2007.

ASQ. 2015. Available at http://asq.org/learn-about-quality/cause-analysis-tools/overview/pareto.html. Accessed 20 Oct 2015.

Baltalden P. Building knowledge for improvement-an introductory guide to the use of FOCUS-PDCA. Nashville: Quality Resource Group, Hospital Corporation of America; 1992.

Campbell RJ. Thinking lean in healthcare. J AHIMA Am Health Informat Manag Assoc. 2009;80(6):40–3; quiz 5–6.

Cima RR, Brown MJ, Hebl JR, Moore R, Rogers JC, Kollengode A, et al. Use of lean and Six Sigma methodology to improve operating room efficiency in a high-volume tertiary-care academic medical center. J Am Coll Surg. 2011;213(1):83–92; discussion 3–4.

de Koning H, Verver JP, van den Heuvel J, Bisgaard S, Does RJ. Lean Six Sigma in healthcare. J Healthcare Q Off Publ Natl Assoc Healthcare Q. 2006;28(2):4–11.

Deming Institute. https://deming.org/. Accessed 10 Oct 2015.

Donabedian A. Evaluating the quality of medical care. Milbank Mem Fund Q. 1966;44 Suppl 3:166–206.

Floriani M. Healthcare Six Sigma project: ED wait times and service quality. 2010. Available at http://www.slideshare.net/mfloriani/healthcare-six-sigma-project. Accessed 19 Oct 2015.

Frankel HL, Crede WB, Topal JE, Roumanis SA, Devlin MW, Foley AB. Use of corporate Six Sigma performance-improvement strategies to reduce incidence of catheter-related bloodstream infections in a surgical ICU. J Am Coll Surg. 2005;201(3):349–58.

Gawande A. The checklist manifesto. New York: Metropolitan Books; 2009.

George M. Lean Six Sigma: combining Six Sigma with lean speed. New York: McGraw-Hill Education; 2002.

Going Lean in Health Care. Cambridge, MA: Institute for Healthcare Improvement; 2005.

Goodridge D, Westhorp G, Rotter T, Dobson R, Bath B. Lean and leadership practices: development of an initial realist program theory. BMC Health Serv Res. 2015;15:362.

Haynes AB, Weiser TG, Berry WR, Lipsitz SR, Breizat AH, Dellinger EP, et al. A surgical safety checklist to reduce morbidity and mortality in a global population. N Engl J Med. 2009;360(5):491–9.

Heijunka. http://leaninstituut.nl/publications/1106/The_Heijunka_Box.pdf. Accessed 26 Oct 15.

HRSA. Developing and implementing a QI plan. 2015. http://www.hrsa.gov/quality/toolbox/methodology/developingandimplementingaqiplan/part2.html. Accessed 17 Oct 2015.

ISQIC. Analyze. In: Bilimoria KY, Yang AD, editors. DMAIC modules. 2014. http://idd.northwestern.edu/elm/isqic/analyze/story.html. Accessed 20 Oct 2015.

ISQIC. Control. In: Bilimoria KY, Yang AD, editors. Available at http://idd.northwestern.edu/elm/isqic/control/story.html. Accessed 21 Oct 2015.

ISQIC. Improve. In: Bilimoria KY, Yang AD, editors. 2014. Available at http://idd.northwestern.edu/elm/isqic/improve/story.html. Accessed 21 Oct 2015.

ISQIC. Measure module. In: Bilimoria KY, Yang AD, editors. DMAIC modules. 2014. Available at: http://idd.northwestern.edu/elm/isqic/measure/story.html.

Kassardjian CD, Williamson ML, van Buskirk DJ, Ernste FC, Hunderfund AN. Residency training: quality improvement projects in neurology residency and fellowship: applying DMAIC methodology. Neurology. 2015;85(2):e7–10.

Knapp S. Lean Six Sigma implementation and organizational culture. Int J Health Care Qual Assur. 2015;28(8):855–63.

Kubiak T, Benbow D. The certified Six Sigma black belt handbook. Milwaukee: ASQ Quality Press; 2005.

Kumar D. Six Sigma best practices. Fort Lauderdale: Ross Publishing, Inc; 2006.

Langley G. The improvement guide: a practical approach to enhancing organizational performance. 2nd ed. San Francisco: Jossey-Bass Publishers; 2009.

Mann D. The missing link: lean leadership. Front Health Serv Manage. 2009;26(1):15–26.

Pyzdek T. The Six Sigma handbook: QA publishing. 1999.

Rhodes RS, Biester TW. Certification and maintenance of certification in surgery. Surg Clin North Am. 2007;87(4):825–36, vi.

Rubin HR, Pronovost P, Diette GB. The advantages and disadvantages of process-based measures of health care quality. Int J Q Health Care J Int Soc Q Health Care ISQua. 2001;13(6):469–74.

Schumacher M. Process improvement overview. 2012. Available at http://www.feinberg.northwestern.edu/research/docs/accr/PIPresentation_8142012.pdf. Accessed 10 Oct 2015.

Schwarz P, Pannes KD, Nathan M, Reimer HJ, Kleespies A, Kuhn N, et al. Lean processes for optimizing OR capacity utilization: prospective analysis before and after implementation of value stream mapping (VSM). Langenbeck's Arch Surg Deutsche Gesellschaft fur Chirurgie. 2011;396(7):1047–53.

Scoville R, Little K. Comparing lean and quality improvement. Cambridge, MA: Institute for Healthcare Improvement; 2014.

Speroff T, O'Connor GT. Study designs for PDSA quality improvement research. Qual Manag Health Care. 2004;13(1):17–32.

Torkki PM, Alho AI, Peltokorpi AV, Torkki MI, Kallio PE. Managing urgent surgery as a process: case study of a trauma center. Int J Technol Assess Health Care. 2006;22(2):255–60.

Waring JJ, Bishop S. Lean healthcare: rhetoric, ritual and resistance. Social Sci Med (1982). 2010;71(7):1332–40.

Zidel T. A lean guide to transforming healthcare: how to implement lean principles in hospitals, medical offices, clinics and other healthcare organizations. Milwaukee: ASQ Quality Press; 2006.

Chapter 3
Measuring Surgical Quality

Andrew M. Ibrahim and Justin B. Dimick

Abstract Improving surgical care requires an in depth understanding of how to measure quality. We are currently witnessing an unprecedented level of investment from payers, policy makers, patient advocacy groups and professional societies to measure the quality of care surgeons provide. Despite the widespread interest in measuring quality, there is little consensus how it should be done. Payers and regulators often target processes of care (e.g. appropriate use of preoperative antibiotics), while surgeons tend to focus on outcomes that are seen as the "bottom line" (e.g. 30-day post-operative mortality rates.) Most recently, numerous stakeholders are advocating for the use of patient reported information (e.g. "How did this operation affect your daily living?")

Abbreviation

PROs   Patient Reported Outcomes

Improving surgical care requires an in depth understanding of how to measure quality. We are currently witnessing an unprecedented level of investment from payers, policy makers, patient advocacy groups and professional societies to measure the quality of care surgeons provide. Despite the widespread interest in measuring quality, there is little consensus how it should be done. Payers and regulators often target

A.M. Ibrahim, MD, MSc
Institute for Healthcare Policy & Innovation, University of Michigan, Ann Arbor, MI, USA

Department of Surgery at Michigan, University Hospitals-Case Medical Center No 2, Cleveland, OH, USA

J.B. Dimick, MD, MPH (✉)
Division of Minimally Invasive Surgery, Center for Healthcare Outcomes and Policy, Ann Arbor, MI, USA

Department of Surgery, University of Michigan, Ann Arbor, MI, USA
e-mail: jdimick@umich.edu

© Springer International Publishing Switzerland 2017   27
R.R. Kelz, S.L. Wong (eds.), *Surgical Quality Improvement*,
Success in Academic Surgery, DOI 10.1007/978-3-319-23356-7_3

processes of care (e.g. appropriate use of preoperative antibiotics), while surgeons tend to focus on outcomes that are seen as the "bottom line" (e.g. 30-day post-operative mortality rates.) Most recently, numerous stakeholders are advocating for the use of patient reported information (e.g. "How did this operation affect your daily living?")

Each of these strategies has benefits and drawbacks that make each different approach appropriate in a specific context. In addition to the goals specified in each context, there are important statistical limitations that can constrain our ability to meaningfully measure quality. This chapter begins with an overview of common measurement approaches and introduces emerging approaches as well. We then review relevant statistical concepts that inform how to choose between each measurement approach.

What Should We Measure? The Structure, Process, Outcomes Framework

The most common framework to measure quality is the "Structure, Process, Outcomes" model described by Donabedian in 1998 (Donabedian 1988). Each component of the model is described below with the benefits and drawbacks of using them in a surgical context (Table 3.1).

Table 3.1 Current approaches to measuring quality in surgery: structure, process outcomes

Type of measure	Example	Benefits	Drawbacks
Structure			
	Hospital Volume	Inexpensive to Measure	May not reflect individual performance
	Intensive Care Unit Staffing	Strong predictor of outcomes for rare, complex operations	Difficult to make actionable
Process			
	Administration of preoperative antibiotic	Straight forward to measure and track	Research still needed to find the best process to target
	Removal of foley by post-operative day 2	Readily Actionable	Adherence does not always translate to better outcomes
Outcomes			
	30 day mortality rate	Strong face-validity with surgeons	Requires large sample sizes to detect meaningful differences
	surgical site infection rates	Reflect the "bottom-line" as seen by most stakeholders	Expensive to collect data for accurate measures

Structure

Structure refers to the measurable elements of a hospital or provider. Examples include hospital size (e.g. number of beds), provider characteristics (e.g. years in training, annual operative volume), or resource availability (e.g. presence of an intensive care unit.) The most attractive aspect of using structure as a quality measure is that the data is highly objective and easily collected. The structure approach to quality was used to describe that higher volume hospitals have improved outcomes for pancreatic resection. While this approach does give important information to compare hospitals broadly, it provides little actionable information for individual improvement within a hospital.

Although the structure approach is helpful to policy makers or payers comparing broadly across multiple hospitals, surgeons pursuing quality improvement within their department or division may find little use for this approach. This approach to measurement does not identify specific pathways for improvement, other than redesigning structures to meet the quality benchmarks. Needless to say, changes to annual volume, hospital beds, or other resources are difficult to make. Many argue that we need to understand why these structural measures are associated with better quality and "export" these details to other facilities. However, an inventory of practices that distinguish high volume from low volume providers, for example, has not been identified.

Process

Process describes the details of care that can be measured. Examples include giving preoperative heparin for thromboembolism prophylaxis or removing an indwelling bladder catheter by post-operative day two to prevent urinary tract infections. Use of process measures has many practical advantages, particularly for local quality improvement initiatives (Bilimoria 2015). First, process measures are straightforward to collect and track. They typically involve a binary variable (e.g. preoperative antibiotics given – yes or no) that does not require risk-adjustment. Second, process measures are highly actionable. While an outlier outcome (e.g. increased surgical site infection rates) may signal a need for quality improvement, a review of adherence to process measures (e.g. preoperative antibiotics, skin decontamination, appropriate bowel prep) directly identifies steps in care that could be improved.

Although process measures are easier to measure and readily actionable, they do have limitations. Because surgical outcomes are often multifactorial, adherence to a process measure does not guarantee an improvement in outcomes. Additionally, because surgical care is complex and so many processes are involved, it can be challenging to identify the best process measure to track and target. As more research develops to find the "right" process measures that best improve outcomes, it will be easier to use this approach to facilitate quality improvement. For departments or hospitals in the early stages of quality improvement, process measures provide an effective and relatively low resource burden approach to begin evaluating and improving performance.

Outcomes

Outcomes represent the end result of care provided. Examples include rates of mortality, complications, or reoperation. A major benefit of this approach is that it enjoys a high degree of clinical-face validity with most surgeons. Unlike approaches to process and structure, however, outcomes are more difficult to measure and therefore require more resources. For example, when comparing process measures between providers one would simply need to determine the, "% of patients who appropriately received perioperative antibiotics." To compare the outcome (i.e. surgical site infection), however, one would need to collect the rate of the event as well as data about the patient specific risk factors for that outcome (e.g. history of surgical site infection, steroid use, type of operation) to allow for fair risk adjustment. Additionally, even with that added information, sufficient volume is needed to avoid Type 1 and Type 2 statistical errors (discussed in detail below.)

While measuring outcomes may be the most challenging and resource intensive, it has been widely adopted by surgical societies, divisions and departments. This likely reflects that surgeons identify with this form of measurement as relevant to practice. Many are optimistic that the burden of collecting data from electronic medical records will become easier and lead to more efficient risk-adjustment models. Even with improved efficiency, however, most outcomes measurement programs in surgery are still constrained by limited sample size (particularly in local quality improvement efforts) to make them useful in detecting differences in quality, as discussed in detail in the next section.

Understanding Statistical Constraints When Measuring Outcomes

Given the complexity of measuring quality using surgical outcomes, and the large number of outcomes measurement programs in surgery, we will devote this section to understanding the statistical nuances of studying variations in surgical outcomes.

All outcome measures will display some variation. Most often, the variation is attributed to the quality of care provided by the hospital or surgeon. There are, however, multiple other reasons for variation to occur related to chance and case-mix that should also be considered. We review them in a surgical context here.

The Role of Chance

When evaluating surgical outcomes, chance can lead to important flaws in inference, known as Type 1 and Type 2 errors. Both of these errors occur more often with low volume procedures (e.g. pancreatic resection) or when with adverse events are

rare (e.g. death after a cholecystectomy.) Because many of the procedures performed by surgeons are relatively rare, or have infrequent adverse events, understanding the role of chance is essential when assessing outcomes.

Type 1 Errors

A Type 1 error occurs when outliers– *good or bad* – are due to chance. Consider,
for example, two surgeons who perform pancreatic surgery. While a death after
pancreatic resection is relatively rare, if the death occurs in a surgeons first five
operations, he or she will inaccurately be labeled with a "20 %" mortality rate.
Similarly, a surgeon who performs five pancreatic resections without a death
will also be misleadingly labeled with a "0 %" mortality rate. The difference in
mortality rates observed between those two surgeons is more likely due to
chance in the setting of low sample size, rather than either exemplary or
substandard care.

The so-called "zero-mortality paradox" observed in a study using Medicare
claims data provides a useful example of a Type 1 error observed at the hospital
level (Dimick and Welch 2008). Researchers reviewed patients undergoing pancreatic resections and identified hospitals with a "0 % mortality" rate for 3 years.
Paradoxically, the following year, those hospitals had mortality rates 30 % higher
than other hospitals. How could that be? On further evaluation it became clear that
those hospitals simply had low volume and "good luck" that led to them inaccurately being labeled high quality. They simply had not performed enough cases yet
to have a bad outcome.

Type 2 Errors

A Type 2 error occurs when differences in quality are not detectable due to limited
sample size. Although Type 2 errors are widely recognized in clinical trials (e.g. the
study was "underpowered"), they are commonly overlooked in surgical quality
improvement efforts. Consider, again, two surgeons who perform pancreatic resections. While there may be real quality differences in the care they provide, it would
be difficult to identify after only 10 operations. After 100 operations, it would
become more clear and with 1000 operations even more so. The ability of increased
sample size to help detect differences between two groups is often referred to "statistical power."

Consider, for example, the *Agency for Healthcare Research and Quality* initiative to use post-operative surgical mortality rates of seven complex operations –
coronary artery bypass graft surgery (CABG), repair of abdominal aortic aneurysm,
pancreatic resection, esophageal resection, pediatric heart surgery, craniotomy, hip
replacement – to identify differences in hospital quality. While principally this
made sense (i.e. hospitals with higher mortality rates for a given procedure are
likely providing lower quality of care), this determination can only be made if there

is enough surgical volume (i.e. enough statistical power) to identify differences. For example, to detect a doubling of mortality among hospitals performing esophageal resections, each would need to complete at least 77 per year. When researchers evaluated all seven of these procedures in the *Nationwide Inpatient Sample*, they found that for 6 of the 7 procedures (all except CABG) the vast majority of hospitals did not perform a minimum case load to detect a doubling of mortality rates (Dimick et al. 2004). In other words, even if there were real differences in quality between hospitals for those operations, low volume would prevent them from being detected.

The Role of Case Mix

Many surgeons confronted with a report identifying them as a poor quality "outlier" argues that their patients are sicker, i.e., that their case-mix is different. Case-mix refers to the type of patients and the type operations being performed. Without question, surgeons and hospitals taking care of sicker patients and doing more complex procedures have a more challenging case-mix that should be acknowledged when we measure outcomes.

The role of case-mix influencing observed outcome rates is most apparent when comparing groups with significant underlying differences. For example, if we wanted to evaluate the mortality rates at a small community hospital performing elective outpatient surgery versus a large tertiary academic center that takes on complex inpatient operations case-mix becomes very important. Even if the same quality of care is provided in both settings, we would still expect a contrast in mortality rates due to differences in patient severity of disease and complexity of the operations performed-- differences in case-mix.

In contrast, when comparing patient populations that are relatively homogenous undergoing similar procedures, accounting for case-mix has less impact. Consider, for example, the mortality rates in the state of New York for patients undergoing coronary artery bypass grafting. The unadjusted rates varied from <1 to 4 %. After adjustment for case-mix, the variation remained the same and was highly correlated (Dimick and Birkmeyer 2008). This should not be surprising because the patients were undergoing the same procedure, had similar underlying diagnoses, and by nature of the disease relatively similar age and health demographics. Thus, the more similar comparison groups are, the less important case-mix becomes in accounting for variation.

For most internal quality improvement efforts, the influence of case-mix on outcomes will be small. Most surgeons' practices' and hospitals systems have little variability year to year in the type of procedures performed or severity of patients being served. While acknowledging variation in case-mix can help establish buy-in from other peer surgeons, minimal resources should be devoted to complex risk-adjustment strategies for local quality improvement projects, unless significant shifts in case-mix are suspected.

Emerging Measurements of Quality in Surgery

While structure, process and outcomes will remain prominent approaches to measuring quality, other measurement strategies are likely to become more visible in the future including patient reported outcomes and surgical video (Table 3.2).

Patient Reported Outcomes

Patient reported outcomes (PROs) include information obtained directly from a patient about their health experience. Examples include patient self-administered questionnaires or focused interviews. They can serve multiple purposes toward measuring and improving the quality of surgical care. First, PROs can further describe the impact of surgery on the patient by soliciting information not captured in our traditional outcomes (e.g. asking about activity levels after a large hernia repair.) Second, PROs may help providers detect when additional interventions are needed (e.g. a patient reported low mobility score prompting a physical therapy evaluation.) Third, PROs may be reported back to individual providers to identify potential patterns of care that could be improved (e.g. provider with consistently high pain scores may re-evaluate his or her post-operative pain regimen.)

Although it is intuitive that we should solicit and incorporate the patient's perspective into how we measure quality and improve care, how to do it well and fairly remains a challenge (Bilimoria et al. 2014). Methodologic issues to be addressed include standardizing questions, integrating the information into already existing medical records and identifying a source of funding for data collection. If PROs are used by payers and regulators to assess providers, then additional research will also be needed to develop appropriate "risk adjustments" for differences in case-mix.

Table 3.2 Emerging measures of quality in surgery: patient reported outcomes, surgical video

Type of measure	Example	Benefits	Drawbacks
Patient Reported Outcomes			
	Generic or disease specific quality of life instruments	Understand outcomes from patient perspective	Instruments and methodology largely unexplored
		Identify gaps in care from a patient perspective	Very burdensome data collection
Surgical Video			
	Video ratings based on skill and technique	Focuses on the quality of the operation, which is understudied	Resource intensive to collect, edit and review surgical video
	Video based peer coaching	Can provide surgeon specific feedback for improvement	Evidence limited to a few procedures (e.g., bariatric surgery)

While methods to obtain PROs are being developed and refined, they will likely have the most uptake initially for operations that our traditional quality measures do not stratify well because they are low volume (e.g. hand surgery) or have low adverse outcome rates (e.g. inguinal hernia repair.)

Use of Surgical Video

While all the previous discussed measurement approaches evaluate what happens to the patient before or after an operation, surgical video uniquely focuses on the operation itself. Because most of our surgical platforms (e.g. laparoscopy, endoscopy) are now fitted with built-in video recording technology, visual data is readily available to surgeons. Early reports in bariatric surgery have been able to correlate an individual surgeon's objective technical skill scores during an operation to his or her patient's post-operative outcomes (Birkmeyer et al. 2013). In doing so, a tremendous amount of interest has been generated in how video data can be used to measure and improve surgical quality.

Multiple possibilities exist for surgical video to be integrated into how we measure and improve surgical quality. For example, individual surgeons are now participating in coaching trials where they watch their own surgical video with a trained peer (i.e. "a coach") to identify where technique can be improved (Greenberg et al. 2015; Hu et al. 2012). In doing so, an entire new range of variables are being identified (e.g. handling to tissue, type of stapler, efficiency of sewing) that may become important measures of quality. In addition to the potential for improving individual surgical quality, if video observed measures are consistently linked to patient outcomes, they may be readily incorporated into surgeon accreditation and board certification. At present, use of surgical video is resource intensive and has only studied for a limited number of procedures.

Choosing the Right Approach to Measure Quality

Recognizing that there are limited resources for quality improvement, it can be difficult to choose where efforts should be prioritized. While there are judgement calls and local limitations about which approach – structure, process, outcomes – can be implemented to measure quality, there are also very real statistical limitations that need to be considered.

Choosing the best measurement approach for quality should take into account the nature of the procedure and our ability to detect differences in what we measure. From a statistical perspective, the more often an event occurs, the easier it is to detect. Therefore, to measure quality for a given procedure we need to ask:

1. How often is the procedure performed? (i.e. Is it high or low volume?)
2. How often does the adverse event occur? (i.e. Is it high or low risk?)

These two questions can guide us to choosing the right approach (Fig. 3.1). Consider the following four categories based on an operations volume and risk.

High Volume, High Risk Procedures

Operations that are high volume and high risk should be evaluated using an outcomes measurement approach. Common examples in this category include bariatric surgery, cardiac surgery, or colectomy. Since these operations are performed commonly and also have relatively frequent adverse outcomes (e.g. colorectal operations surgical site infection rates as high as 30 %) there is enough statistical power to detect differences in *outcomes*.

High Volume, Low Risk Procedures

Process measures and patient reported outcomes are best utilized for procedures that are high volume but have low risk. A common example is the inguinal hernia repair. Although it is one the most common general surgery procedures performed, complications in outcomes are rare (e.g. 30 day mortality <1 %). Differences in patient reported outcomes (e.g. post-operative pain, quality of life measures) or adherence to process measures (e.g. appropriate use of perioperative beta-blocker medication) occur more frequently and therefore more useful when looking for differences in quality.

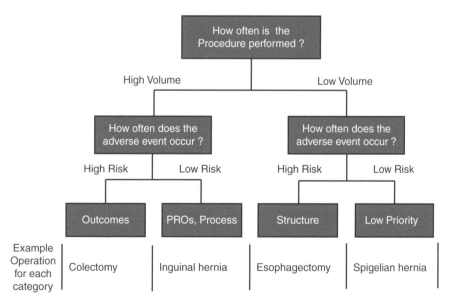

Fig. 3.1 Choosing between different approaches to measuring surgical quality

Low Volume, High Risk Procedures

When procedures are low volume and high risk, structure is the most appropriate approach to evaluating quality. Esophageal resection is an illustrative example. Although it is an operation with a high complication rate, it is performed relatively rarely such that we do not have enough statistical power to detect meaningful differences in either outcomes or process measures. To date, our best evidence now supports structure elements (e.g. operative volume) as the best empiric predictor of quality and future performance (Birkmeyer et al. 2006).

Low Volume, Low Risk Procedures

Finally there are procedures that fit neither outcomes, process or structure approaches because they are low volume and low risk. Operations in this category (e.g. Spigelian hernia) should be given low priority for quality improvement initiatives in favor of operations mentioned above that are more common or have more risk.

Additional Considerations for Measuring Outcomes

Measuring outcomes has the most face-validity with surgeons interested in quality improvement, but is also the most challenging to do fairly. As described above, variation in observed outcomes may be highly influenced by case-mix and chance that can be partially accounted for with different statistical techniques including risk-adjustment and reliability-adjustment.

Risk Adjustment

Risk adjustment can help account for variation that is due to differences in case-mix. This is most frequently done with a multivariable logistic regression model that uses measurable differences in patients (e.g. age, gender, race) to adjust their risk for an outcome. How much "adjustment" is needed depends on the underlying differences between the groups being compared. Although there is eagerness to include as many as 21 "adjustment variables", for procedure specific comparisons (i.e. comparing patients undergoing the same operation) as few as 5 variables can be used to provide the same amount of adjustment (Dimick et al. 2010). This is important to identify because the differences in resources required to collect 5 versus 21 data points about each patient can be significant burden. Again, for internal quality improvement efforts where there is low variability in case-mix, risk-adjustment should not be prioritized.

Reliability Adjustment

Reliability adjustment can help evaluate if the variation observed is due to true differences in performance or instead "statistical noise" caused by low sample size. This approach is more complicated, but briefly uses hierarchical modeling and Bayesian methods to average an individual surgeon outcome rate with the outcomes rate of all the surgeons combined in a weighted fashion based on volume. In this model, a surgeon who has performed zero operations is assumed to be whatever is the average rate of all the surgeon in that group until he or she performed enough operations to stratify themselves are either a high or low performer. The weighted nature of this model results in lower volume surgeons being "adjusted" closer to the mean. While this reliability adjustment can prevent inaccurate labelling of low volume providers as high or low outliers, it also results in a "shrinkage" in the observed variation making it more difficult to detect differences in quality that exist.

Conclusion

Understanding how to measure quality in surgery is necessary for performance improvement. The role of chance when sample sizes are small is often overlooked and can mislabel surgeons inaccurately into high and low providers. Adjustments for case-mix, although available, are resource intensive and for many local quality improvement efforts not necessary. If case-mix adjustments are applied, every effort should be taken to stream line them to a limited number of variables. In addition to our current measures of process, structure and outcomes, new sources of data such patient reported outcomes and surgical video will likely be integrated into the mainstream of quality assessment. Finally, and most importantly, measurement of quality is necessary, but not sufficient for quality improvement. All efforts to measure performance should be coupled focused interventions to improve care.

References

Bilimoria KY. Facilitating quality improvement: pushing the pendulum back toward process measures. JAMA. 2015;314(13):1333–4.

Bilimoria KY, Cella D, Butt Z. Current challenges in using patient-reported outcomes for surgical care and performance measurement: everybody wants to hear from the patient, but are we ready to listen? JAMA Surg. 2014;149(6):505–6.

Birkmeyer JD, Dimick JB, Staiger DO. Operative mortality and procedure volume as predictors of subsequent hospital performance. Ann Surg. 2006;243(3):411–7.

Birkmeyer JD, Finks JF, O'Reilly A, et al. Surgical skill and complication rates after bariatric surgery. N Engl J Med. 2013;369(15):1434–42.

Dimick JB, Birkmeyer JD. Ranking hospitals on surgical quality: does risk-adjustment always matter? J Am Coll Surg. 2008;207(3):347–51.

Dimick JB, Welch HG. The zero mortality paradox in surgery. J Am Coll Surg. 2008; 206(1):13–6.

Dimick JB, Welch HG, Birkmeyer JD. Surgical mortality as an indicator of hospital quality: the problem with small sample size. JAMA. 2004;292(7):847–51.

Dimick JB, Osborne NH, Hall BL, Ko CY, Birkmeyer JD. Risk adjustment for comparing hospital quality with surgery: how many variables are needed? J Am Coll Surg. 2010;210(4):503–8.

Donabedian A. The quality of care. How can it be assessed? JAMA. 1988;260(12):1743–8.

Greenberg CC, Ghousseini HN, Pavuluri Quamme SR, Beasley HL, Wiegmann DA. Surgical coaching for individual performance improvement. Ann Surg. 2015;261(1):32–4.

Hu YY, Peyre SE, Arriaga AF, et al. Postgame analysis: using video-based coaching for continuous professional development. J Am Coll Surg. 2012;214(1):115–24.

Chapter 4
Are You Capable of Providing High Quality Care?

Affan Umer and Scott Ellner

Abstract Quality improvement (QI) initiatives have intensified in the healthcare workplace with only a nascent understanding of the definition of quality in healthcare. As physicians, we adhere to the Hippocratic aphorism of "do no harm" and therefore, often delude ourselves into believing that we are functioning at the top of our clinical capacity and knowledge for the benefit of our patients. It is undeniable that nearly all physicians want to do what is best for their patients. However, maximizing the potential for improved outcomes can prove challenging.

Understanding Quality in Healthcare

Quality improvement (QI) initiatives have intensified in the healthcare workplace with only a nascent understanding of the definition of quality in healthcare. As physicians, we adhere to the Hippocratic aphorism of "do no harm" and therefore, often delude ourselves into believing that we are functioning at the top of our clinical capacity and knowledge for the benefit of our patients. It is undeniable that nearly all physicians want to do what is best for their patients. However, maximizing the potential for improved outcomes can prove challenging.

Physicians often fail to comprehend the significance of the components of quality represented by structure and process and moreover, the link to the resultant outcomes is often indirect, at best. The unfortunate result is an ambiguity and occasional ambivalence about QI. Therefore, it should come as no surprise that individual physicians feel burdened and, perhaps instinctively resistant to sharing responsibility for QI.

Over the last few decades, medical science, knowledge and technology has advanced at such an unprecedented rate, so as to overshadow the growth in parallel concepts such as safety, quality and human factors (Waring et al. 2016). Such factors

A. Umer, MD
General Surgery, UConn Health Center, Farmington, CT, USA

S. Ellner, DO, MHCM, FACS (✉)
General Surgery & Trauma Surgery, Saint Francis Hospital and Medical Center, Hartford, CT, USA
e-mail: SEllner@stfranciscare.org

© Springer International Publishing Switzerland 2017
R.R. Kelz, S.L. Wong (eds.), *Surgical Quality Improvement*,
Success in Academic Surgery, DOI 10.1007/978-3-319-23356-7_4

are often overlooked until medical errors occurred and forced participants to address the issues. To improve patient care, we know that a broadened approach to viewing the clinical environment is warranted. In his outline of the anatomy of the healthcare system, Dr. David Burton describes a healthcare delivery system of craftsmanship, the quality of which is strictly tethered to the ability and intelligence of human providers (https://www.healthcatalyst.com/anatomy-healthcare-delivery-model-transform-care). Accordingly, for QI strategies to take root and be effective, they need ownership and acceptance from individuals in the surgical community.

The Institute of Medicine (IOM) defines quality in healthcare as a multi-dimensional concept (http://www.nationalacademies.org/hmd/~/media/Files/Report%20Files/2001/Crossing-the-Quality-Chasm/Quality%20Chasm%202001%20%20report%20brief.pdf) with six key points:

- (a) Health care should be efficient. Patients should get the care they need; consequently avoid underuse of health care resources and (b) patients should need the care they receive; avoiding unnecessary interventions.
- Care should be provided safely,
- It should be provided in a timely manner,
- It should be patient centered,
- It should be delivered equitably,
- And it should be delivered efficiently. As to avoid waste.

Understanding the plurality of quality is essential to navigating its complexity and these key points provide the necessary framework to achieve clarity in action. Though we need to be wary, these dimensions exist to understand quality as a whole and not fragment it (Beattie et al. 2012).

Taking Responsibility for Quality Improvement

Approximately 14–17% of surgical admissions result in an adverse event (Thomas et al. 2000; Anderson et al. 2013). Errors in non-operative management are more frequently encountered then operative errors (Anderson et al. 2013). Mastering surgical technique is only part of the continuum that embodies quality surgical care. Our responsibility for the wellbeing of the patient begins from admission and extends to the point where the patient completely recovers from the surgical insult. In order to execute this obligation effectively, we need to create a culture of safety and quality. Surgeons are natural leaders in the OR, that is why it is critical that surgeons take utmost responsibility and extend their leadership role to non-operative quarters.

Surgical quality improvement is still in nascent phase and while the industry builds high reliability systems that minimize human errors we must simultaneously build highly reliable teams to minimize risk. Appropriate behaviors, actions, attitudes and cognition must align in this team and do so repeatedly to guarantee a desired outcome. Effective communication is integral for quality initiatives to succeed. A proficient surgeon must communicate his intentions and coordinate with team members. The team members in turn must be able to speak freely, voicing any concerns, fears or disagreements not only for the common goal of patient safety but also from the perspective of efficiency. Fostering this culture creates behavioral safety nets, so if and when an adverse event occurs, any member of the team can react, within capacity, to first limit harm and then identify avenues for improvement. Similarly, identifying processes that are too costly, increasingly time consuming, are distracting from patient care and have potential for automation or standardization are all avenues for quality improvement.

Theoretically, it may seem convenient for a surgeon to assume the role of a leader but leadership is a complex clinical function and our training rarely affords us the luxury of its mastery. We must be proficient clinicians and simultaneously possess knowledge of organizational structure, managerial agendas, workflow streams and be actively engaged with hospital administration and bureaucracy. It also requires a rudimentary understanding of human psychology. In essence, physician leaders should possess a good foundation of emotional intelligence in order to be effective leaders. Especially with the transition to a value-based purchasing model of healthcare, it is imperative that we embrace this duality in roles. Our reimbursements are tied to high quality care which means we need to be invested in QI efforts. We need to forego comfort seeking and rather develop problem sensing approaches. Simple measures such as implementing the surgical checklist, ensuring proper handovers during transitions of care and procedural timeouts can prevent unnecessary and fatal adverse events. Integrating QI strategies often requires re-organizing the present work force, re-visiting their roles and responsibilities, establishing effective interdisciplinary communication, and reiterating evidence based strategies as the rule.

The need for quality, however, shouldn't burden the workforce as such an approach may generate resistance to change. Hayes et al. comments that in order to achieve true and sustainable improvement in outcomes, we must, at all levels of the system, understand and aim to embed a "work smarter, not harder" approach and limit the workload, including that associated with improvement-related activities, on those charged with delivering care (Hayes et al. 2015). Unfortunately, QI efforts are rarely subject to such meticulous thought, especially when they are forced down by an administrative hierarchy. Surgeons, however, understand their dominion; they stand at the crossroads where policy and practice intersect. This gives us a more practical vantage point to inspire change and navigate around difficulties in our path. We are essential to the future of quality in healthcare. Gerald W. Peskin echoes this sentiment stating that the quality of surgical care cannot improve unless we harness the knowledge and creative energy of surgeons for the purpose of redesigning the intricate process that constitutes modern health care (Peskin 2002).

Quality and the Surgeon of the Future

We are in the midst of a transformational era of consumerism in healthcare. This movement has led to calls for increased patient autonomy, greater accountability and transparency which includes reporting outcomes publicly. Subsequently, surgeons are faced with the challenges of being measured and rated more than ever.

Such scrutiny comes from external oversight bodies, medical societies and third parties who are peripherally invested in the business of healthcare quality. How we react to these difficulties will ultimately define how relevant we are to the future of our specialty. Rifat Latifi critically evaluates the evolving landscape in surgery and concludes that the surgeon of the future needs to be patient-centered, disease-focused, technology-driven, and team-focused but above all he must be adaptable (Latifi et al. 2015) to a changing landscape geared toward value-based care.

Surgeons no longer work or act alone. Interdisciplinary collaboration is integral to quality care. Surgical teams, consulting subspecialties, physical therapists, pain specialists, nutritional experts and discharge coordinators all are essential to improving surgical outcomes. An adaptable surgeon is at the center of this collaboration. Adaptability further requires intervening to support communication, responding appropriately to external and internal pressures and constantly dealing with the uncertainty and ambiguity in structure, process and outcomes measures.

Historically, one of the limitations for quality improvement was the lack of reliable data that measured quality outcomes and our ability to produce valuable conclusions from it. Fortunately, such barriers no longer exist and a plethora of disease, specialty and outcome specific data is available to us. Risk adjusted and validated data such as that from the American College of Surgeons' National Surgical Quality Improvement Program allows us to measure and benchmark surgical outcomes regionally through collaboratives and nationally. The surgeon of the future must be data-oriented in order to bring about sustainable change. Any reliable data when presented effectively can guide care for patients, prevent adverse events, enhance interdisciplinary collaboration and most importantly – for a leader – it can make the difference needed to change a culture in an organization on the journey to provide care of the highest quality.

Patient-Centered Care and Quality

Traditionally, surgical specialties focused on attaining meticulous skill and expansive knowledge of anatomy and disease to deliver effective care. These basic tenets of our field are necessary for technical excellence and hold very much true to date but over the years the definition of what constitutes effective care has changed. The new paradigm of quality care requires engaging with patients on a more personal level, taking into account their cultural, religious and socioeconomic differences, and presenting them with relevant clinical and non-clinical data to allow for high quality, informed patient- centered decision making.

Shared decision-making is embedded in the Affordable Care Act, and allows patients to become involved in decisions and to choose less invasive interventions or more conservative options (Stacey et al. 2011). This has the potential for avoiding unnecessary interventions which might otherwise be more aligned with physician rather than patient preference. A 2011 Cochrane collaborative review found patients who had decision aids were more knowledgeable with greater risk perception and had less internal conflict regarding healthcare decisions (Stacey et al. 2011). These avenues have potential for increasing patient satisfaction, improving their compliance with treatments and both indirectly and directly reducing healthcare costs. Surgeons must relinquish their paternalistic approach and adopt strategies that are more considerate of patient needs. We must train ourselves to show high degrees of empathy and emotional intelligence in order to develop deeper insight into the anxieties and uncertainties that inflict our patients. Avedis Donabedian, a prominent healthcare quality theorist, emphasized that quality of care encompasses not only technical excellence but what holds equal merit is the humanity and manner with which care is delivered (Donabedian 1968). Ultimately there will be a point where despite all precautions an undesired outcome will occur, and the only thing that might salvage this precarious situation is time spent by clinicians forging a relationship with the patient. Our humanistic side is often diluted by the overbearing complexity of our profession, but if allowed to shine through, can nurture the progress in QI we wish to see.

Fostering traits such as emotional intelligence are also beneficial in dealing with difficult patients, co-workers and administrators alike. Inspirational leadership, teamwork, conflict resolution, effective communication, are all skills that are enhanced under the domain of emotional intelligence.

Conclusions

The quality movement in healthcare will continue to test new waters, see what works and how well. Surgeons should be effective contributors to these efforts to catalyze progress. The future will be very empowering for the engaged surgeon. The most important consequence of our pursuit of QI is probably not the organizational change we are striving for but the change and development in attitudes and behaviors of individuals.

References

Anderson O, Davis R, Hanna GB, Vincent CA. Surgical adverse events: a systematic review. Am J Surg. 2013;206(2):253–62.

Beattie M, Shepherd A, Howieson B. Do the Institute of Medicine's (IOM's) dimensions of quality capture the current meaning of quality in health care?–An integrative review. J Res Nurs. 2012;18:288–304.

Donabedian A. Promoting quality through evaluating the process of patient care. Med Care. 1968;6(3):181–202.

Hayes CW, Batalden PB, Goldmann D. A 'work smarter, not harder' approach to improving healthcare quality. BMJ Qual Saf. 2015;24(2):100–2.

http://www.nationalacademies.org/hmd/~/media/Files/Report%20Files/2001/Crossing-the-Quality-Chasm/Quality%20Chasm%202001%20%20report%20brief.pdf. Accessed 14 Feb 2016.

https://www.healthcatalyst.com/anatomy-healthcare-delivery-model-transform-care. Accessed 22 Feb 2016.

Latifi R, Dudrick SJ, Merrell RC. The new surgeon: patient-centered, disease-focused, technology-driven, and team-oriented. In: Technological advances in surgery, trauma and critical care. New York: Springer; 2015. p. 3–8.

Peskin GW. Quality care in surgery. Arch Surg. 2002;137(1):13–4.

Stacey D, Bennett CL, Barry MJ, Col NF, Eden KB, Holmes-Rovner M, et al. Decision aids for people facing health treatment or screening decisions. Cochrane Database Syst Rev. 2011;10:CD001431.

Thomas EJ, Studdert DM, Burstin HR, Orav EJ, Zeena T, Williams EJ, et al. Incidence and types of adverse events and negligent care in Utah and Colorado. Med Care. 2000;38:261–71.

Waring J, Allen D, Braithwaite J, Sandall J. Healthcare quality and safety: a review of policy, practice and research. Sociol Health Illn. 2016;38(2):181–97.

Chapter 5
Surgical Quality Improvement: Local Quality Improvement

Ira L. Leeds and Elizabeth C. Wick

Abstract The quality movement has dramatically changed both the practice and perception of healthcare over the last 30 years. In surgery, the unique details of any particular patient's case may have made comparative quality reporting and benchmarking more challenging, but these obstacles should not let the surgical care of patients to be omitted from quality movement. The variation in outcomes following standardized surgical procedures has been recognized for many years. The Northern New England Cardiovascular Disease study group first reported regional variations in mortality following coronary artery bypass procedures that were attributable to different processes of care rather than underlying patient factors in 1996 (O'Connor et al. JAMA 275:841–846, 1996). Since then, a plethora of national and regional collaboratives have been organized to identify outperforming and underperforming institutions in an effort to highlight best practices for improving patient outcomes. Some of the most successful registry-based quality improvement efforts include the Society for Vascular Surgery Vascular Quality Index, Washington state's Surgical Care and Outcomes Assessment Program, the Michigan Surgical Quality Collaborative, and the Tennessee Surgical Quality Collaborative. These collaboratives have identified important areas of improvement for enhanced patient outcomes and have disseminated their findings into everyday surgical practice (Englesbe et al. Ann Surg 252:514–519, 2010; Guillamondegui et al. J Am Coll Surg 214:709–714, 2012; Kalish et al. J Vasc Surg 60:1238–1246, 2014; Simianu et al. Ann Surg 260:533–538, 2014).

I.L. Leeds, MD, MBA
Department of Surgery, The Johns Hopkins Hospital, Baltimore, MD, USA

E.C. Wick, MD (✉)
Department of Surgery, University of California, San Francisco, CA, USA
e-mail: ewick1@jhmi.edu

© Springer International Publishing Switzerland 2017
R.R. Kelz, S.L. Wong (eds.), *Surgical Quality Improvement,*
Success in Academic Surgery, DOI 10.1007/978-3-319-23356-7_5

Key Points
- Surgical quality improvement ultimately requires implementation of the best evidence-based findings at each local institution
- Successfully implementing quality improvement locally requires the appropriate administrative structures and processes
- Inter-disciplinary collaborative relationships at the frontline are essential for success
- Management of local quality improvement structures and processes can be a meaningful and important commitment for early-career surgical faculty

Introduction

The quality movement has dramatically changed both the practice and perception of healthcare over the last 30 years. In surgery, the unique details of any particular patient's case may have made comparative quality reporting and benchmarking more challenging, but these obstacles should not let the surgical care of patients to be omitted from quality movement. The variation in outcomes following standardized surgical procedures has been recognized for many years. The Northern New England Cardiovascular Disease study group first reported regional variations in mortality following coronary artery bypass procedures that were attributable to different processes of care rather than underlying patient factors in 1996 (O'Connor et al. 1996). Since then, a plethora of national and regional collaboratives have been organized to identify outperforming and underperforming institutions in an effort to highlight best practices for improving patient outcomes. Some of the most successful registry-based quality improvement efforts include the Society for Vascular Surgery Vascular Quality Index, Washington state's Surgical Care and Outcomes Assessment Program, the Michigan Surgical Quality Collaborative, and the Tennessee Surgical Quality Collaborative. These collaboratives have identified important areas of improvement for enhanced patient outcomes and have disseminated their findings into everyday surgical practice (Englesbe et al. 2010; Guillamondegui et al. 2012; Kalish et al. 2014; Simianu et al. 2014).

However, national and regional approaches for surgical quality improvement have their limitations. On one hand, these efforts represent a unique method for compiling the large datasets and diverse patient populations needed for the statistical analyses that have demonstrated that practice variation matters. Without these registry-based quality improvement initiatives, there would not be the belief amongst surgeons that it is possible to continually improve and there would be fewer best practices on which to act to improve patient outcomes. Conversely, these same quality improvement efforts are necessarily limited in the change they can effect on the individual healthcare institution or individual practitioner.

While national quality registries may dominate much of the public discussion of surgical quality improvement efforts, the day-to-day work of quality improvement continues in every institution in the country through the committed work of health-care practitioners incrementally improving the care patients receive. These local efforts are ultimately how surgical quality improvement will directly affect patients, and reducing the variability in local quality improvement implementation is likely as important as the discovery of new best practice recommendations for improving patient outcomes (Fig. 5.1).

The difficulty of local implementation of quality improvement initiatives is routinely underestimated, and there are many factors that can contribute to the likelihood of implementation success (e.g., institutional size, administrative support, employee engagement, validity of data, financial and human resources, etc.). However, many of these obstacles to effective local quality improvement are intrinsic features of institution and are often difficult, if not impossible, to change except with large organizational shifts in priorities. Rather than focusing on inherent obstacles to quality improvement, we have found that there adapting to extant institutional environment is possible with the rational design of quality improvement administrative structures and processes. This chapter will highlight practices that we have found useful for implementing local quality improvement initiatives as well as how to use those practices to manage an academic career in local quality improvement.

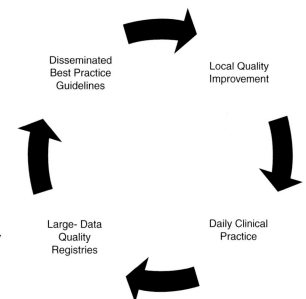

Fig. 5.1 National-local cyclic quality improvement. This diagram demonstrates the cyclical relationship between national/regional quality improvement efforts and local quality improvement. Daily clinical practice provides the data for aggregated quality registries, from which best practice recommendations are made, and then depend on local quality improvement efforts to reach the case of patients

Disseminated
Best Practice
Guidelines

Local Quality
Improvement

Large- Data
Quality
Registries

Daily Clinical
Practice

Designing for Local Quality Improvement

The practice of healthcare invariably occurs in a dynamic system. Disease patterns, patient needs, payer relationships, and regulatory requirements are constantly changing. Such an exciting, ever-changing environment is what draws many into clinical care, but this phenomenon has also made it difficult to easily export quality improvement models from other industries. Adopting the high reliability processes of the aviation industry has often been encouraged in healthcare (Weick and Sutcliffe 2001), but aviation is highly standardized with limited intrinsic variability. The concept of high reliability organizations is critical for aviation because critical events are so rare but also inevitably catastrophic if not avoided. In contrast, healthcare has a high degree of intrinsic variability due to the unique nature of continually changing patient factors and unpredictability of disease presentation. Errors happen in healthcare practice routinely and often do not cause measurable patient harm (Institute of Medicine 2000).

The following sections describe important tenets of designing a structure and process for local quality improvement in the context of an ever-changing, dynamic healthcare system.

Building a Culture of Change

The goal of surgical quality improvement is not to develop a single, rigid set of processes that categorically reduces risks to patients and improves outcomes. Instead, surgical quality improvement – particularly at the local level – should be focused on fostering a culture of change where quality improvement efforts are developed, disseminated, and reassessed in an iterative fashion.

One of the most promising models for promoting a culture of change and facilitating a structured process for healthcare quality improvement at the local level has been Comprehensive Unit-based Safety Programs (CUSPs). The CUSP model has been shown to be effective at reducing bloodstream infections in variety of medical specialties and diverse care environments (Berenholtz et al. 2011, 2014; Pronovost et al. 2006; Sexton et al. 2011; Sawyer et al. 2010). Most recently, CUSP has been used for perioperative surgical quality improvement with substantial decreases observed in surgical site infection rates among early adopters and increased perioperative team engagement (Hicks et al. 2014; Wick et al. 2012). The tenets of CUSP are based on a 5-step process (Table 5.1) that heavily emphasize engagement of key stakeholders, front-line education, and a preoccupation with identifying the next quality improvement need.

The CUSP model is based on recognition that the individual clinical unit is ultimately where quality improvement must occur and that, alone, frontline providers are not able to overcome institutional barriers. It acknowledges the inherent limitations of national best practices and focuses on empowering front-line workers to perform an iterative quality monitoring and action program based on local

Table 5.1 Comprehensive unit-based safety program (CUSP) components

Component	Implementation example
1. Science of safety education	Introductory talk to explain the approach to addressing safety at a local level
2. Staff safety assessment	Two-question survey to team members
3. Senior executive partnership	Senior executive attendance at CUSP meetings, assisting with system-wide barriers
4. Learning from defects	Uses structured defect-learning tool
5. Implement teamwork and communication tools	Review unit-level safety data, develop local quality improvement initiative, address hazards

Adapted from Wick et al. (2012)

circumstances and partners them with a senior hospital executive to bridge the executive-frontline divide and instill joint accountability toward meaningful improvement. The advantages of such an approach appear to be high levels of front-line engagement (Hicks et al. 2014; Wick et al. 2012). The CUSP approach fosters "small wins." For example, one perioperative CUSP team, quickly identified a long-standing lack of hot water in scrub sinks. On investigation, the maintenance department had not been empowered to order the missing part to restore the hot water but through the partnering CUSP senior executive this was addressed and the hot water was restored. Feeling empowered to make suggestions about other areas of safety and quality, frontline providers then gave direct feedback about observed lapses in sterile technique during the latter half of colorectal procedures that led to the addition of a second set of clean instruments for closure (unpublished data, Charles Bosk, Ph.D.). While neither of these practices have made it into national guidelines documents, grassroots efforts such as these performed at the unit level have led to both high levels of provider compliance and improvements in quality metrics.

Communicating Quality

As the CUSP model described above notes with its emphasis on provider education and teamwork tools, much of the success seen with local quality improvement is attributed to intrinsic or self-motivation of front-line workers. Getting support from clinical providers is less about obtaining top-down administrative decree and more suited to positive engagement through open, clear communication.

Healthcare institutions are beginning to understand the importance of communicating local quality improvement expectations to front-line providers. At Johns Hopkins Medicine, one of the simplest strategies has been the circulation of an internal monthly electronic newsletter to all faculty and staff that openly addresses strengths and opportunities for improvement within the institution's quality efforts. Past issues have addressed the results of an institution-wide safety culture assessment and standardizing processes for a new electronic medical record platform.

More recently, our institution has also taken the novel step of increasing dissemination and transparency of unit-based quality metrics. The Johns Hopkins Armstrong Institute for Patient Safety and Quality has developed a Patient Safety and Quality Dashboard that allows any clinical provider to immediately view unit-level data for federally-reported core measures, hospital epidemiology compliance, and patient satisfaction survey results. Such dissemination of quality data allows for unit-to-unit comparisons and helps frame conversation about planned quality interventions. It has effectively turned every front-line provider into a local quality improvement champion.

A related form of quality improvement feedback has also been growing with the increasing influence of hospital rankings. While we believe that current methods used to generate rankings have a number of flaws and may not be appropriate for a patient looking for a healthcare institution, they are useful as a form of externally validated quality local quality improvement feedback. Specifically, hospital rankings are helpful in highlighting quality metrics for which a particular healthcare institution underperforms. If the local quality improvement team believes the particular quality metric in question to be important, rankings data provides a useful benchmark and framing device to use for discussing potential quality improvement interventions.

Emory University Hospital in Atlanta, Georgia was very successful with this approach over the last 5 years using the University HealthSystem Consortium's (UHC) quality rankings. The institution was historically ranked in the top half of 118 participating academic medical centers. After an internal team recognized the shared goals of the UHC metrics and those of the institution, a multi-year plan was enacted to align hospital operations with the UHC quality metrics. Since then, the hospital has ranked in the top ten member institutions since 2012. Emory's chief quality officer noted that the success was due to utilizing the rankings to mobilize a culture of staff commitment and targeted new services that focused on specific healthcare quality goals (Christenbury 2013).

Management of Quality Data

An institution's knowledge about the quality of care delivered is limited by how that quality is measured. Measurement of quality is not easy. The limitations of existing quality metrics for comparative analysis is an ongoing major area of investigation in outcomes research (Birkmeyer et al. 2004). Although quality metric *reporting* is controversial, consensus exists around the need to measure quality internally. An important first step to measuring quality is the development an internal data management process that standardizes and facilitates the collection of quality measures as well as their analysis.

Many of the current electronic medical records platforms employed by hospitals do not include robust quality reporting processes. In current practice, it is not unusual for one component of a patient's electronic medical record to interface with clinical units, further quality data to come from administrative billing records, and a third silo of data being housed in ancillary departments such as hospital epidemiology. Developing a comprehensive sense of an institution's overall quality improvement needs from such a disparate data environment is almost impossible.

One approach to streamlining quality analytics has been the development of comprehensive data repositories of all clinical, administrative, and research data for a healthcare institution. Emory University Hospital is known to a have single clinical data warehouse that has been used to centralize all clinical data for enhanced analysis of its externally reported quality metrics (Shin et al. 2014). The Ohio State University Medical Center has also been a major proponent of comprehensive data warehousing for both clinical and financial applications (Kamal et al. 2010). Typically, these systems have large upfront setup costs that have prevented widespread adoption, but proponents have argued that ease of each individual analytic exercise makes the approach justifiable over a longer time horizon.

With the rise of quality reporting as a major driver of new healthcare information technology acquisitions by hospitals, newer electronic medical record platforms are beginning to directly integrate quality metric analytics. Epic Systems Corporation's operational intelligence product Cogito™ is an option offered with its current electronic medical record platform. These platform add-ons can increase the cost of an institution's electronic medical record contract and typically require high level hospital executive-level support for inclusion.

Both of the approaches highlighted above represent a high degree of interoperability that is required between clinical and administrative data sources within a hospital to support effective used of data for quality improvement. Securing an effective data management plan for quality measures and their analysis should be a priority for internal quality champions. Ultimately, this need for good data management will likely extend beyond the scope of an institution's quality improvement efforts and require a substantial degree of diplomacy at the highest levels of the institution to ensure the appropriate data management structures are in place.

Making Your Career in Local Quality Improvement

The administrative processes and structures described above rarely occur by chance within a healthcare institution. These must be carefully selected for and designed by internal quality champions who understand both the administrative and clinical demands of quality improvement efforts.

We strongly believe that these roles cannot be easily performed by non-clinicians. There are subtleties in local quality improvement that must be managed by clinical care providers. With respect to managing a culture of change, front-line healthcare workers must lead these efforts to avoid alienating their peer providers targeted by these interventions. Communication with clinicians must also be done in a way that is sensitive to language of direct patient care and providers' intrinsic motivations. Finally, data management efforts that skew away from data related to direct clinical care are unlikely to capture the critical bedside quality information needed to inform and monitor good quality improvement interventions.

Surgical faculty are well-poised to be the clinical champions leading local quality improvement efforts. Their practice takes them to myriad departments within institutions including perioperative care, critical care units, laboratory medicine, inpatient care, and hospital-based outpatient clinics. Their regular interaction with all types of frontline providers (nurses, technicians, residents, physicians from consulting services, etc.) fosters cross-disciplinary collaboration. Perhaps most importantly, the recent interest in surgeon-specific variation in surgical quality (Birkmeyer et al. 2013) and expected increased scrutiny of surgical outcomes further incentivizes an active role by surgeons in local quality improvement efforts.

To be successful, committed surgeons should consider formal training in quality improvement. This can be accomplished through formal degree granting programs like Master of Business Administration (MBA) or Master of Hospital Administration (MHA) or through intensive, focused coursework on quality improvement offered through national organizations like the Institute for Healthcare Improvement (IHI), Intermountain Healthcare, and the National Patient Safety Foundation (NPSF) among others. Ultimately, to be a surgical leader in this arena clinicians need to have well-developed leadership skills in addition to being well-versed in the key attributes and methodology of process improvement.

The likely greatest hurdle to local quality improvement is the lack of funded roles offered by healthcare institutions. The importance of quality metrics for hospitals' financial reimbursements is helping to address this issue, but junior faculty may not be able to expect compensation for every quality role offered to them. However, junior faculty member desiring to pursue this course should begin to establish an independent and collaborative track record of successful quality improvement work. Such efforts can even be started as a surgical trainee. Promising projects to work on are those that have the attention of senior administrators while also not being insurmountable. Engagement and progress will help build one's institutional reputation and translate to long-term academic career success in this expanding field.

Conclusion

All quality improvement efforts do not require national headlines and book tours. The quality work that will most likely affect individual patients is done locally at virtually every healthcare institution. Being successful at a local quality improvement first requires a strategic analysis at the structures and processes already in place and a plan for addressing any deficiencies. With that perspective, one can build out an appropriate platform of quality monitoring and pilot interventions. Dramatically improving the quality of care of patients at the local level can be more difficult than one might expect, but success can come with both intrinsic and extrinsic rewards for an academic surgeon.

References

Berenholtz SM, Pham JC, Thompson DA, Needham DM, Lubomski LH, Hyzy RC, et al. Collaborative cohort study of an intervention to reduce ventilator-associated pneumonia in the intensive care unit. Infect Control Hosp Epidemiol. 2011;32(4):305–14.

Berenholtz SM, Lubomski LH, Weeks K, Goeschel CA, Marsteller JA, Pham JC, et al. Eliminating central line-associated bloodstream infections: a national patient safety imperative. Infect Control Hosp Epidemiol. 2014;35(1):56–62.

Birkmeyer JD, Dimick JB, Birkmeyer NJ. Measuring the quality of surgical care: structure, process, or outcomes? J Am Coll Surg. 2004;198(4):626–32.

Birkmeyer JD, Finks JF, O'Reilly A, Oerline M, Carlin AM, Nunn AR, et al. Surgical skill and complication rates after bariatric surgery. N Engl J Med. 2013;369(15):1434–42.

Christenbury J. University HealthSystem Consortium ranks two Emory hospitals in top 10 nationally for quality achievements, 2013. 9 Aug 2015. Available from: http://news.emory.edu/stories/2013/10/2013_uhc_rankings/.

Englesbe MJ, Brooks L, Kubus J, Luchtefeld M, Lynch J, Senagore A, et al. A statewide assessment of surgical site infection following colectomy: the role of oral antibiotics. Ann Surg. 2010;252(3):514–9. Pubmed Central PMCID: 2997819, discussion 9–20.

Guillamondegui OD, Gunter OL, Hines L, Martin BJ, Gibson W, Clarke PC, et al. Using the National Surgical Quality Improvement Program and the Tennessee Surgical Quality Collaborative to improve surgical outcomes. J Am Coll Surg. 2012;214(4):709–14. discussion 14–6.

Hicks CW, Rosen M, Hobson DB, Ko C, Wick EC. Improving safety and quality of care with enhanced teamwork through operating room briefings. JAMA surg. 2014;149(8):863–8.

Institute of Medicine. To err is human: building a safer health system. Washington, DC: National Academy of Sciences; 2000.

Kalish JA, Farber A, Homa K, Trinidad M, Beck A, Davies MG, et al. Factors associated with surgical site infection after lower extremity bypass in the Society for Vascular Surgery (SVS) Vascular Quality Initiative (VQI). J Vasc Surg. 2014;60(5):1238–46.

Kamal J, Liu J, Ostrander M, Santangelo J, Dyta R, Rogers P, et al. Information warehouse – a comprehensive informatics platform for business, clinical, and research applications. AMIA Annu Symp Proc/AMIA Symp AMIA Symp. 2010;2010:452–6. Pubmed Central PMCID: 3041278.

O'Connor GT, Plume SK, Olmstead EM, Morton JR, Maloney CT, Nugent WC, et al. A regional intervention to improve the hospital mortality associated with coronary artery bypass graft surgery. The Northern New England Cardiovascular Disease Study Group. JAMA. 1996;275(11):841–6.

Pronovost P, Needham D, Berenholtz S, Sinopoli D, Chu H, Cosgrove S, et al. An intervention to decrease catheter-related bloodstream infections in the ICU. N Engl J Med. 2006;355(26):2725–32.

Sawyer M, Weeks K, Goeschel CA, Thompson DA, Berenholtz SM, Marsteller JA, et al. Using evidence, rigorous measurement, and collaboration to eliminate central catheter-associated bloodstream infections. Crit Care Med. 2010;38(8 Suppl):S292–8.

Sexton JB, Berenholtz SM, Goeschel CA, Watson SR, Holzmueller CG, Thompson DA, et al. Assessing and improving safety climate in a large cohort of intensive care units. Crit Care Med. 2011;39(5):934–9.

Shin SY, Kim WS, Lee JH. Characteristics desired in clinical data warehouse for biomedical research. Healthc Inform Res. 2014;20(2):109–16. Pubmed Central PMCID: 4030054.

Simianu VV, Bastawrous AL, Billingham RP, Farrokhi ET, Fichera A, Herzig DO, et al. Addressing the appropriateness of elective colon resection for diverticulitis: a report from the SCOAP CERTAIN collaborative. Ann Surg. 2014;260(3):533–8. Pubmed Central PMCID: 4160115, discussion 8–9.

Weick K, Sutcliffe K. Managing the unexpected: assuring high performance in an age of complexity. San Francisco: Jossey-Bass; 2001.

Wick EC, Hobson DB, Bennett JL, Demski R, Maragakis L, Gearhart SL, et al. Implementation of a surgical comprehensive unit-based safety program to reduce surgical site infections. J Am Coll Surg. 2012;215(2):193–200.

Chapter 6
How to Address a Quality Problem

Brandyn D. Lau and Elliott R. Haut

Abstract For quality improvement (QI) projects, the Translating Research into Practice (TRiP) framework is an ideal model for developing and addressing topics locally (see Fig. 6.1) (Pronovost et al. BMJ 337:a1714, 2008). The TRiP framework is a four-step process that evaluates best practices with the goal of creating strategies for implementation at a local level. Using high-quality evidence, the TRiP framework utilizes multidisciplinary collaboration to incorporate knowledge translation for broader dissemination of knowledge into practice. Each step focuses on systems of care rather than care of individual patients with engagement of multidisciplinary teams to assume ownership of the QI project. Finally, this framework encourages adaptation so that the QI intervention can meet the culture of the implementing group when expanded regionally or nationally (Pronovost et al. BMJ 337:a1714, 2008). At the Johns Hopkins Hospital, we have successfully utilized this framework to reduce central line-associated blood stream infections (Pronovost et al. BMJ 340:c309, 2010) and improve prescription of risk-appropriate venous thromboembolism (VTE) prophylaxis (Streiff et al. BMJ 344:e3935, 2012). For this purposes of this chapter we will give examples of these successful interventions, though each step can be applied to meet different quality improvement goals.

Translating Research into Practice (TRiP)

For quality improvement (QI) projects, the Translating Research into Practice (TRiP) framework is an ideal model for developing and addressing topics locally (see Fig. 6.1) (Pronovost et al. 2008). The TRiP framework is a four-step process that evaluates best practices with the goal of creating strategies for implementation at a local level. Using high-quality evidence, the TRiP framework utilizes

B.D. Lau, MPH, CPH • E.R. Haut, MD, PhD, FACS (✉)
Division of Acute Care Surgery, Department of Surgery, Johns Hopkins University School of Medicine, Baltimore, MD, USA

Department of Health Policy and Management, The Johns Hopkins University Bloomberg School of Public Health, Baltimore, MD, USA

The Armstrong Institute for Patient Safety and Quality, Johns Hopkins Medicine, Baltimore, MD, USA
e-mail: ehaut1@jhmi.edu

Fig. 6.1 Four Step
Translating Research into
Practice (TRiP) framework
for quality improvement
(Pronovost et al. 2008)

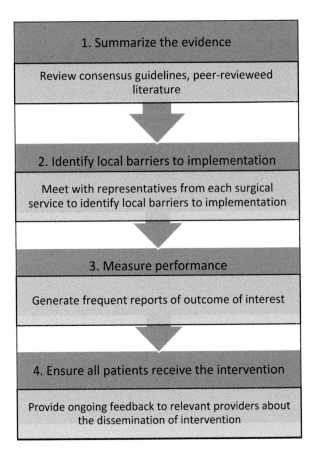

multidisciplinary collaboration to incorporate knowledge translation for broader dissemination of knowledge into practice. Each step focuses on systems of care rather than care of individual patients with engagement of multidisciplinary teams to assume ownership of the QI project. Finally, this framework encourages adaptation so that the QI intervention can meet the culture of the implementing group when expanded regionally or nationally (Pronovost et al. 2008). At the Johns Hopkins Hospital, we have successfully utilized this framework to reduce central line-associated blood stream infections (Pronovost et al. 2010) and improve prescription of risk-appropriate venous thromboembolism (VTE) prophylaxis (Streiff et al. 2012). For this purposes of this chapter we will give examples of these successful interventions, though each step can be applied to meet different quality improvement goals.

Identifying and Defining a Quality Topic

The first step to addressing a quality problem is to identify and comprehensively define the topic of interest. There are nearly as many ways to identify a quality topic as there are quality topics to address. There are two primary pathways for identifying potential quality topics: external benchmarking and internal audits.

External benchmarking for topic identification requires comparable data from one or more other institutions. A common example of this methodology is comparison of data related from your institution to aggregated data reported in national registries. Some national registries applicable to surgical benchmarking include the American College of Surgeons' National Surgical Quality Improvement Program (ACS NSQIP), the University HealthSystem Consortium (UHC), and the National Trauma Data Bank (NTDB). The benefits of these large national data registries include standardization of metrics across hospital settings and providing sufficiently large samples of patients from which to establish a benchmark. However, these registries often lack the granularity to clearly define root causes for differences in reported outcomes across settings, potentially limiting the ability to determine the reason for differential outcomes and possible approaches to fix the problem.

Internal audits for topic identification are often less standardized or generalizable, but frequently offer the greatest opportunity for improvement within organizations. Internal audits often begin with internal discussion and/or observations which may arise from Morbidity and Mortality conferences, patient safety and adverse event reporting, or simply anecdotal evidence. The critical first step is to examine data for the proposed problem before starting to remedy a problem that may not truly exist. Frontline providers including residents, physician assistants, nurse practitioners, and bedside nurses often provide the most valuable input about potential opportunities for quality improvement that can fix a process and therefore improve the outcome. These frontline providers are most directly associated with the quality of care that patients receive, and have valuable input about the culture and practices of care.

Defining the topic or quality problem requires consideration of all of the potential contributing factors. While some problems may be fairly direct, more complex multifactorial problems may require a structured approach to identify numerous possible root causes. One example of a structured approach to identify causes to a specific problem is to construct an Ishikawa Diagram, also known as a fishbone diagram (see Fig. 6.2a), to identify both upstream and downstream contributors to a specific problem of interest. This formal process enables the investigative team to conceptualize the problem and identify key individuals and stakeholder groups who can contribute to the characterization and remedy.

For the example of improving VTE prevention practices for surgical patients that we will provide in this chapter, we adopted a hybrid approach. First, we sought to understand how our institution performed internally regarding the prescription of risk-appropriate VTE prophylaxis for surgical patients (Streiff et al. 2012; Haut et al. 2012; Monn et al. 2013; Aboagye et al. 2013). An internal audit of the surgical services at The Johns Hopkins Hospital in 2005 found that only 33 % of 322 randomly selected surgical patients were prescribed VTE prophylaxis consistent with the American College of Chest Physicians (ACCP) guidelines. After exploring the root causes and applying a series of targeted interventions, we compared our performance with other hospitals using publicly reported data (Johnbull et al. 2014; Kardooni et al. 2008). These findings represented a deficit in quality that affects patient safety (Goldhaber et al. 2004) and institutional reputation (Johnbull et al. 2014; Bilimoria et al. 2013), and presented a clear opportunity for a QI project.

Fig. 6.2 (a) Ishikawa
diagram example of root
causes for a common QI
problem. (b) Example
Ishikawa diagram for missing
consent forms at the time of
surgery (Garonzik-Wang
et al. 2013)

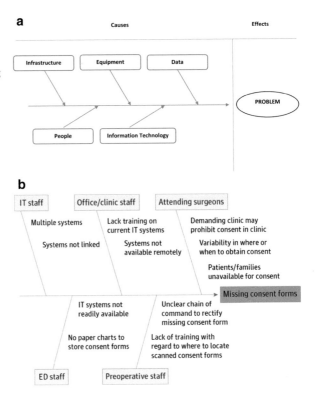

Assemble a Multidisciplinary Team

Gone are the days of having a team of surgeons fix problems in radiology and
pathology. Critical to the mission of addressing a surgical QI problem is assembling a multidisciplinary team consisting of all relevant stakeholders who supply
input for the problem to be fixed. The contemporary approach to building a multidisciplinary team is to consider all required expertise needed to address a defined
quality problem. If medication prescription or administration is a critical component, a member of the pharmacy team would provide another valuable perspective.
In addition to clinical input, other types of individuals can provide valuable expertise and knowledge. For specific projects, clinicians and researchers may be the
most recognizable members of the team; however, many roles are often overlooked
when developing a true transdisciplinary team. Librarians/informationists are
extremely helpful when identifying literature that is relevant to the topic of interest.
Similarly, biostatisticians provide important methodological expertise regarding
the analytic plan for evaluating your quality problem while social psychologists
and/or human factors engineers may be valuable for assisting with implementation
and dissemination.

In our example of improving VTE prophylaxis prescribing habits, we required multidisciplinary input to achieve the "Five Rights" to aid in decision making. These include providing the right information, to the right person, in the right format, through the right channel, at the right time in the workflow (Campbell 2013). Our VTE Collaborative team is comprised of a surgeon, hematologist, nurses, pharmacists, a clinical information, and quality and safety clinical researchers. Each member of the team provides critical input on clinical effectiveness of medication regimens for a variety of risk levels to determine the right information. From a human factors approach, physicians and informaticians determined that prescribers who wrote admission orders for the patient were the right person and was universally agreed that the electronic health record (EHR) system would be the right channel. It was determined that the right format would be a mandatory decision support tool that requires prescribers to complete a short risk assessment linked to a VTE order set and that the right time to is during the initial admission and subsequent transfer processes when providers are assessing patients for a variety of conditions (Streiff et al. 2012).

Summarize the Evidence

After the topic of interest has been identified, the first step within the TRiP framework is to summarize the evidence. If it's a problem at one hospital, it likely exists at other hospitals and it is important to understand what is known about the topic of interest and what evidence gaps exist. Succinct summaries of the evidence can be found in clinical practice guidelines, systematic reviews and meta-analyses. Reviewing these sources can be supplemented with a literature review to capture more recent evidence or studies that are more specific to the topic of interest.

In our example of improving VTE prophylaxis use, we first reviewed the clinical guidelines for VTE prevention from the ACCP and determined that the practices pertinent to VTE prevention were: (1) identify service-specific patient risk factors for VTE and bleeding; (2) stratify patients into VTE risk categories; (3) prescribe corresponding prophylaxis recommendations; and (4) recommend treatment alternatives for patients with contraindications to pharmacologic prophylaxis.

Identify Local Barriers to Complying with the Evidence

All QI efforts are undertaken with the implicit assumption that we, as healthcare providers, want to provide the highest quality of care to our patients and that we must bridge the gap between evidence and practice. Having input from a multidisciplinary team that includes all contributors to delivering care regarding your topic of interest is critical to understand what specific barriers exist and how to overcome them.

As part of an Accreditation Council for Graduate Medical Education (ACGME)-required resident QI project, one resident team focused on missing consent forms on the day of surgery and used a mixed methods approach to define the magnitude of the problem and identify specific barriers to having a completed consent form. In this particular analysis where 66 % of patients were missing signed consent forms, multiple contributing factors played a part including technological failures, poor communication among clinical staff, and physician workflow challenges (Garonzik-Wang et al. 2013). These challenges were summarized in an Ishikawa diagram to identify target options to facilitate intervention (see Fig. 6.2b).

Within the example of VTE prophylaxis prescription, conversations with the care team led to the discovery that practice was not standardized both in terms of clinical workflow and determination of appropriate care. To standardize practice, we initially developed six service-specific paper-based order sets to accommodate the major clinical services (e.g., surgery, trauma, orthopedics, medicine); however, there were many barriers to implementation. Clinicians found it was time-intensive to locate and complete a paper form, and it was not part of their normal order entry workflow in the presence of a computerized provider order entry (CPOE) system. Consequently, this led to the development of a computerized VTE risk assessment tool that made VTE risk-assessment, coupled with decision support to recommend the correct prophylaxis regimen, a mandatory part of the admission and transfer process (Streiff et al. 2012).

Measure Performance

"If you can't measure it, you can't change it." One fundamental aspect of quality improvement is the measurement of the change in quality of care after interventions have been implemented. In order to determine this trajectory, it is imperative that a clear, standardized outcome of interest be defined. This outcome should be measurable before and after your intervention has been implemented. In the era of EHR, vast amounts of data are collected and are able to be reported electronically. Every effort should be made to identify standardized variables that are captured in the EHR that directly or indirectly evaluate the quality of care that patients receive. While there is an initial investment of time in refining the variables for reporting, this effort pays great dividends when reporting outcomes for ongoing quality monitoring. With data comes the power to make change.

Within our example of VTE prevention, our team initially focused on measuring the process of care by tracking compliance with suggested VTE prophylaxis. The primary process measures were proportions of patients risk stratified and ordered risk-appropriate VTE prophylaxis (both dichotomous variables). We developed a HIPAA-compliant Web-based VTE database to facilitate data analysis and generate reports of VTE prophylaxis performance on an institutional, departmental, divisional, service, and individual clinical provider level (Streiff et al. 2012). As a result of this method of measurement, we have been able to assess changes in practice on both a hospital-wide level, and for specific services and patient populations (Haut et al.

2012; Monn et al. 2013; Aboagye et al. 2013; Zeidan et al. 2013; Lau et al. 2015a). Furthermore, we have used this ability to measure to provide continuous feedback to frontline providers to sustain and further improve practice (Lau et al. 2015b, c, 2016).

Ensure All Patients Receive the Intervention

The problem that is defined likely exists for other patient populations at other hospitals. Successful QI interventions should be shared broadly to ensure that all patients receive the highest quality of care possible. First, it is important to consider how a QI solution could be modified and expanded to other floors, departments, and hospitals to be as generalizable as possible. Second, consider the communication strategy for disseminating findings, describing the QI problem, intervention, and methods. A well-written manuscript will describe in sufficient detail how others may adapt and implement your intervention to meet their own needs (Holzmueller and Pronovost 2013).

For improving VTE prophylaxis prescription, we re-examined the literature and found that active computer-based systems are much better than education alone to increase guideline compliance and adequate prophylaxis (Lau and Haut 2014). Another barrier regarding the paper order sets expressed consistently by front-line physicians was the belief that their patients were different and the paper tools were too general and not applicable to their population. To respond to this concern, we developed 16 different service-specific modules in conjunction with clinicians to address each patient population's unique risks and contraindications.

Improving Culture and Learning from Mistakes

The comprehensive unit based safety program (CUSP) has demonstrated dramatic improvements in surgical safety culture (Timmel et al. 2010). As part of CUSP, a senior executive partners with a group or unit and actively participates as a member of the quality improvement team. The team works to identify and learn from one defect each month, which is brought to the attention of department and hospital leadership. The goal is to focus intently on specific and actionable issues, and work to improve practice (Pronovost et al. 2006).

Sustain Quality Improvements

The purpose of QI interventions are to modify and sustain behavioral change that are associated with improved patient outcomes (Fan et al. 2010). A solution that relies on human input or manual data collection rarely allows for ongoing, long-term, sustained improvement or scalability. A byproduct of a successful intervention is the generation of new knowledge about what works, and what does not, to facilitate behavioral modification for other QI targets. Ongoing efforts should consider the effects of QI interventions, including increased risk of harm, the use of new technological interventions, and the synthesis of the growing body of literature related to the topic of interest.

Opening Pandora's Box

At the Johns Hopkins Hospital, through a series of multifaceted QI interventions, we assured that 98 % of surgical patients were prescribed risk-appropriate VTE prophylaxis (Lau et al. 2015c). During the process of reaching this high-reliability level, we discovered that many doses of VTE prophylaxis are never administered to patients (Shermock et al. 2013; Haut et al. 2015) and that patients who receive more diagnostic studies for VTE are more likely to have an event diagnosed (Pierce et al. 2008), whereby biasing our publicly reported quality measures (Johnbull et al. 2014; Bilimoria et al. 2013; Haut and Pronovost 2011). Quality improvement is a multi-level cycle, and no problem might ever truly be fixed. However, the reward in addressing a QI problem is making a measurable difference in the quality of care that patients receive.

References

Aboagye JK, Lau BD, Schneider EB, Streiff MB, Haut ER. Linking processes and outcomes: a key strategy to prevent and report harm from venous thromboembolism in surgical patients. JAMA Surg. 2013;148(3):299–300. doi:10.1001/jamasurg.2013.1400.

Bilimoria KY, Chung J, Ju MH, et al. Evaluation of surveillance bias and the validity of the venous thromboembolism quality measure. JAMA. 2013;310(14):1482–9. doi:10.1001/jama.2013.280048.

Campbell R. The five "rights" of clinical decision support. J AHIMA. 2013;84(10):42–7; quiz 48.

Fan E, Laupacis A, Pronovost PJ, Guyatt GH, Needham DM. How to use an article about quality improvement. JAMA. 2010;304(20):2279–87. doi:10.1001/jama.2010.1692.

Garonzik-Wang JM, Brat G, Salazar JH, et al. Missing consent forms in the preoperative area: a single-center assessment of the scope of the problem and its downstream effects. JAMA Surg. 2013;148(9):886–9. doi:10.1001/jamasurg.2013.354.

Goldhaber SZ, Tapson VF, DVT FREE Steering Committee. A prospective registry of 5,451 patients with ultrasound-confirmed deep vein thrombosis. Am J Cardiol. 2004;93(2):259–62.

Haut ER, Pronovost PJ. Surveillance bias in outcomes reporting. JAMA. 2011;305(23):2462–3.

Haut ER, Lau BD, Kraenzlin FS, et al. Improved prophylaxis and decreased preventable harm with a mandatory computerized clinical decision support tool for venous thromboembolism (VTE) prophylaxis in trauma patients. Arch Surg. 2012;10(147):901–7.

Haut ER, Lau BD, Kraus PS, et al. Preventability of hospital-acquired venous thromboembolism. JAMA Surg. 2015;150(9):912. doi:10.1001/jamasurg.2015.1340.

Holzmueller CG, Pronovost PJ. Organising a manuscript reporting quality improvement or patient safety research. BMJ Qual Saf. 2013;22(9):777–85. doi:10.1136/bmjqs-2012-001603.

Johnbull EA, Lau BD, Schneider EB, Streiff MB, Haut ER. No association between hospital-reported perioperative venous thromboembolism prophylaxis and outcome rates in publicly reported data. JAMA Surg. 2014;149(4):400–1. doi:10.1001/jamasurg.2013.4935.

Kardooni S, Haut ER, Chang DC, et al. Hazards of benchmarking complications with the National Trauma Data Bank: numerators in search of denominators. J Trauma. 2008;64(2):273–7. doi:10.1097/TA.0b013e31816335ae; discussion 277–9.

Lau BD, Haut ER. Practices to prevent venous thromboembolism: a brief review. BMJ Qual Saf. 2014;23(3):187–95.

Lau BD, Haider AH, Streiff MB, et al. Eliminating health care disparities with mandatory clinical decision support: the venous thromboembolism (VTE) example. Med Care. 2015a;53(1):18–24. doi:10.1097/MLR.0000000000000251.

Lau BD, Streiff MB, Pronovost PJ, Haider AH, Efron DT, Haut ER. Attending physician performance measure scores and resident physicians' ordering practices. JAMA Surg. 2015b;150(8):813–4. doi:10.1001/jamasurg.2015.0891.

Lau BD, Arnaoutakis GA, Streiff MB, et al. Individualized performance feedback to surgical residents improves appropriate venous thromboembolism (VTE) prophylaxis prescription and reduces potentially preventable VTE: a prospective cohort study. Ann Surg. 2015c. [Epub ahead of print]. http://www.ncbi.nlm.nih.gov/pubmed/26649586.

Lau BD, Streiff MB, Hobson DB, et al. Beneficial "Halo Effects" of surgical resident performance feedback. J Surg Res. 2016. http://www.ncbi.nlm.nih.gov/pubmed/26649586 .

Monn MF, Haut ER, Lau BD, et al. Is venous thromboembolism in colorectal surgery patients preventable or inevitable: one institution's experience. J Am Coll Surg. 2013;216(3):395–401.

Pierce CA, Haut ER, Kardooni S, et al. Surveillance bias and deep vein thrombosis in the national trauma data bank: the more we look, the more we find. J Trauma. 2008;64(4):932–6. doi:10.1097/TA.0b013e318166b808; discussion 936–7.

Pronovost PJ, Berenholtz SM, Goeschel CA, et al. Creating high reliability in health care organizations. Health Serv Res. 2006;41(4 Pt 2):1599–617. doi: HESR567 [pii].

Pronovost PJ, Berenholtz SM, Needham DM. Translating evidence into practice: a model for large scale knowledge translation. BMJ. 2008;337:a1714. doi:10.1136/bmj.a1714.

Pronovost PJ, Goeschel CA, Colantuoni E, et al. Sustaining reductions in catheter related blood-stream infections in Michigan intensive care units: observational study. BMJ. 2010;340:c309. doi:10.1136/bmj.c309.

Shermock KM, Lau BD, Haut ER, et al. Patterns of non-administration of ordered doses of venous thromboembolism prophylaxis: implications for novel intervention strategies. PLoS One. 2013;8(6):e66311. doi:10.1371/journal.pone.0066311.

Streiff MB, Carolan H, Hobson DB, et al. Lessons from the Johns Hopkins Multi-Disciplinary Venous Thromboembolism (VTE) Prevention Collaborative. BMJ. 2012;344:e3935.

Timmel J, Kent PS, Holzmueller CG, Paine L, Schulick RD, Pronovost PJ. Impact of the Comprehensive Unit-based Safety Program (CUSP) on safety culture in a surgical inpatient unit. Jt Comm J Qual Patient Saf. 2010;36(6):252–60.

Zeidan AM, Streiff MB, Lau BD, et al. Impact of a venous thromboembolism prophylaxis "smart order set": improved compliance, fewer events. Am J Hematol. 2013;88(7):545–9. doi:10.1002/ajh.23450.

Chapter 7
Barriers and Pitfalls in Quality Improvement

Ryan D. Macht and David McAneny

Abstract Quality improvement (QI) is complex and often challenging. While the aim of QI is to create meaningful and sustained improvements in patient care, projects routinely fall short of this goal. These failures are typically due to several frequently encountered pitfalls that may occur throughout the QI process. The intent of this chapter is to examine some of the common reasons for QI project failure and to determine how these problems can be avoided. We shall use examples from our own experiences, incorporating lessons learned when overcoming barriers.

Those familiar with quality improvement (QI) projects can attest that this work may be a daunting experience. Improvement science incorporates both technical elements and adaptive challenges, including human behavior and organizational culture. Difficulties in either aspect can derail even the most promising project. While the science of healthcare QI has been formalized only relatively recently, these principles and the corresponding failures are not new. Perhaps the most infamous example involves the nineteenth century Hungarian physician, Ignaz Semmelweis, who had attributed marked differences in maternal mortality from puerperal fever to hand washing practices and antiseptic techniques in separate clinics (Gillies 2005). Even with compelling data and simple, sensible technical elements of handwashing that would have reduced deadly infections, he was unable to overcome the adaptive challenges of garnering support from other physicians for his revolutionary idea. He ultimately failed to change traditional behavior. Because of his persistence, Semmelweis was ostracized by the medical community, dismissed from his hospital, and eventually committed to a mental institution, where he died shortly after being beaten by guards.

While successful QI projects often receive notoriety and glory, both institutionally and in publications, it may be the failed efforts from which we can learn the most. Surgeons routinely evaluate complications at Morbidity and Mortality conferences to analyze and understand adverse outcomes in order to prevent

R.D. Macht, MD • D. McAneny, MD, FACS (✉)
Department of Surgery, Boston University School of Medicine, Boston Medical Center,
Boston, MA, USA
e-mail: david.mcaneny@bmc.org

© Springer International Publishing Switzerland 2017
R.R. Kelz, S.L. Wong (eds.), *Surgical Quality Improvement*,
Success in Academic Surgery, DOI 10.1007/978-3-319-23356-7_7

them from recurring. The intent of this chapter is to similarly examine common reasons why QI projects fail, as well as how these lapses can be avoided. We shall use failures from our own experiences, incorporating lessons learned and how we overcame these challenges. The discussion of common QI barriers and pitfalls will hopefully allow the reader to improve quality without encountering many of the struggles that we and others, like Semmelweis, have previously endured.

Pitfall #1: Failure to Choose an Appropriate Project and Scope

Choosing the ideal quality improvement project aim and area of focus is not an obvious or simple endeavor. When initially engaging in surgical QI, the number of issues and potential projects will be overwhelming. Selecting an inappropriate project can lead to results that are either disappointing or convey little impact. An early victory is also beneficial in that failure can adversely affect the credibility of and trust in the QI group; success breeds success. Therefore, it is best to seek "low hanging fruit" in inaugural projects. That may involve a discrete priority within the department, a clear opportunity to improve (no place to go but up), or an effort that will not require extensive staff and resources. Metrics from high fidelity clinical databases, such as the American College of Surgeons National Surgical Quality Improvement Program (NSQIP), can be used to identify areas with the greatest opportunities for improvement. For example, our initial NSQIP report in 2009 revealed disappointing data in both pulmonary and venous thromboembolism (VTE) complications. Rather than simultaneously tackling both of these major problems, we dealt with them in succession. The pulmonary program, designated as "ICOUGH" (vide infra), generated excitement among nursing staff and created early successes (Cassidy et al. 2013). We focused on ICOUGH with a singular purpose, postponing the VTE project until we had sufficient support and institutional standing to begin a new effort.

We recently embarked upon another project with the intent of decreasing readmissions to the Surgical Intensive Care Unit (SICU). We selected three key areas of focus: developing objective SICU admission/discharge criteria, standardizing handoffs among several groups of clinicians, and creating a large multidisciplinary team to conduct daily rounds on patients for 48 h after transfer out of the SICU. It soon became apparent that the scope of the project was too great, despite the value of the effort. Initial enthusiasm about a project can lead to goals that either are too lofty, involve too many groups of people, or require changes in too many areas. It is essential to respect the limits of a team and to design a program that is realistic. A pilot project's scope and allocated resources may expand and become more comprehensive over time. However, a strategy based on imposing additional work on clinicians who are already quite busy is not one to predicate success upon.

Pitfall #2: Failure to *ADOPT* What Has Worked Elsewhere

One of the advantages of QI work is that the majority of challenges are common to other hospitals and clinicians. A common mistake is to try to "reinvent the wheel," without investigating what has succeeded or failed elsewhere. For example, catheter associated urinary tract infection (CAUTI) is a pervasive complication, and several organizations have reduced the incidence of this infection in various settings. We charged a task force to address CAUTI several years ago. One of the urologists on the team had hoped to draw upon the experience of surgeons with whom she had worked at the Veterans Administration Medical Center, where a nurse-driven protocol had reduced the likelihood of CAUTIs among orthopedic patients (Uberoi et al. 2013). However, other committee members disagreed and instead focused on physician and nurse education. The CAUTI rates did not substantially change, and so the nurse-driven protocol is being entertained once again.

While innovative approaches are often favored, possibly due to the desire to publish novel or unique projects, sometimes the easiest tactic with the best chance for success is what has already been effective elsewhere. In addition to a standard literature search, several resources provide details about QI successes, including NSQIP archives or the BMJ Quality Improvement Reports database (BMJ 2015).

Pitfall #3: Failure to *ADAPT* What has Worked Elsewhere

At the other end of the spectrum of pitfall #2 is not modifying what has worked elsewhere to fit the intrinsic circumstances and environmental context of the organization. Before starting any QI project, it is important to consider the local situation and determine the optimal setting and timing for the work. For example, if several other projects have been recently implemented on a particular unit, staff may be challenged to manage priorities that compete for time and attention. In fact, numerous concomitant changes can be overwhelming. Similarly, if a particular surgical service has not previously welcomed QI projects, it may be better to pilot an intervention with another service and then disseminate the practices more broadly once established.

Understanding the environmental context is critical at the conception and introduction of a project. While we encourage using other institutions' successful approaches, these should also suit the local strengths and obstacles of personnel and resources. A "one size fits all" approach to QI is rarely effective. Failing to modify QI projects to the local environment is a primary reason why initiatives that succeed in one context may be ineffective when scaled to various settings, a concept known as the "Iron Law" (Perla et al. 2015). Perla describes checklists as a recent example of this phenomenon. While initial studies associated perioperative checklists with significant declines in deaths and complications, a similar benefit was not realized when implemented on a larger-scale in Ontario, Canada (Urbach et al. 2014). The disparate results among studies are likely multifactorial, but mandating that rigid protocols be universally applied, without factoring how best to locally implement or adapt them, is likely a flawed philosophy.

Our staff dealt with perioperative checklist-related fatigue and variable compliance as the number of mandatory – and often redundant or unnecessary – items exploded for each patient. The local context was not entirely appreciated during the mass implementation, and, not surprisingly, the checklists were inconsistently obeyed. We resolved this matter by identifying essential steps, reducing the number of points, and coordinating timing of checklist segments based upon the flow of perioperative care. Properly designed checklists should engender communication rather than promote dissent among the ranks.

Pitfall #4: Failure to Address and Measure Technical Aspects of a Project

While some assume that QI work does not need a formal methodological approach, successful QI initiatives do follow the tenets of improvement science. The technical aspects of this discipline have been described in greater detail in other chapters, but they are important to emphasize because the lack of structure for design, implementation, and measurement is a frequent cause of failure. This often occurs when clinicians assume they can simply "wing it".

After receiving reports about errors in communication and management during the transition of care between the Emergency Department and the surgical services, we sought to improve this process with a handoff checklist among residents in each department. However, we initially focused only on resident communication without using a structured framework and tools like process mapping to identify other causes of error. While communication among residents improved, the errors persisted because only one aspect of the transition of care had been addressed. Many different quality and implementation frameworks are available, each with advantages and disadvantages. While no single system is ideal for all situations, we believe it is imperative to use one of these disciplined approaches for each project, regardless of the size and scope of the initial aim.

Another potential technical pitfall is designing a project without selecting appropriate metrics to monitor. In surgery, while we are usually more interested in outcome measures such as complication rates, these events may be infrequent and unsuitable for short-term surveillance. Instead, process measures that are proxies for outcomes may be more enlightening. For example, in a project to reduce colorectal surgical site infections (SSIs), metrics about aspects of SSI reduction bundle compliance may be more facile and immediately meaningful than semiannual NSQIP reports. Relevant and timely data are needed to provide valuable feedback to both staff and the QI team (Bradley et al. 2004).

Pitfall #5: Failure to Assemble a Well-Rounded Project Team

A strong team with diverse perspectives consistently accomplishes QI initiatives more successfully than even the most motivated individual. As a result, time spent assembling the components of the team is well rewarded. A common pitfall when building a team is not enlisting frontline staff, including residents. We learned this lesson when attacking the rate of vascular surgery infections. The attending surgeons and QI staff initially focused on surgical instruments and modifying sterilizing procedures, with little effect. The team then engaged frontline staff from both the operating room and the surgery floors. The collective insight introduced new ideas about perioperative hygiene and wound care that were later associated with improved outcomes. Involving frontline members from a project's inception increases cooperation among those who are actually responsible for implementing clinical changes.

A successful QI team includes participants with a variety of talents and departmental interests. A sound team building strategy considers strengths and weaknesses of potential members that match the needs of the project, as opposed to randomly soliciting volunteers. In fact, the composition of effective teams can be retained for future projects, as they are more likely to be successful than novices (O'Neill 2011). As encountered with the vascular SSI initiative, the deliberate assembly of a larger group cultivated a team spirit, especially in the operating room. When stronger interpersonal relationships develop, team members perceive a greater shared pride and stake in patients' well-being and outcomes. Of course, the selection or natural declaration of solid leaders is paramount. An ideal team will promote leaders, foster shared interests, and possess institutional credibility.

Pitfall#6: Failure to Appreciate "Adaptive Challenges" in Behavior and Culture

One of the most difficult aspects of QI involves modification of human behavior and organizational culture to accomplish a particular aim. While it is fair to assume that all healthcare providers desire what is best for their patients, it is naïve to assume this attitude alone will sustain abrupt changes in behavior and practice. A common QI pitfall involves focusing only on the technical elements of a project, without addressing the adaptive challenges to assure widespread acceptance among those who will be most affected by the changes. This shortcoming especially disenfranchises frontline staff, and an attentive QI team must recognize and remedy that vulnerability. These human and cultural deficiencies, referred to as adaptive challenges, are pervasive in QI and "can only be addressed through changes in people's priorities, beliefs, habits, and loyalties" (Pronovost 2011). This is perhaps the most daunting and yet most gratifying facet of QI endeavors.

Pronovost has proposed several methods to confront adaptive challenges, but one that resonates is to "surface the real and perceived losses" for those resisting behavioral change (Pronovost 2011). This reaction was captured during the implementation of an Enhanced Recovery After Surgery (ERAS) protocol. Despite our group's record of successful QI programs, some adaptive challenges of this comprehensive project have still been troublesome. While we had anticipated resistance to certain changes invoked by ERAS, we could not have expected that the most controversial practice would involve the transfer of patients from the recovery room to the surgery floor in wheelchairs rather than on stretchers. We had conceived this gesture as a powerful cue to encourage early mobilization of patients after operations. However, the proposal encountered considerable resistance from the recovery room staff. While the initial complaints were logistical (e.g., insufficient space or a lack of enough wheelchairs), we soon realized that perceived losses truly fueled this sentiment. The staff believed that their professional discretion had become compromised and that changes were made without their opinions. We initiated a weekly ERAS huddle in the recovery room to provide a forum for voicing concerns and to instantly address conflicts and outstanding issues. Engagement in the initiative has subsequently improved.

Another adaptive challenge presents when an organization's culture is not conducive to QI. This culture is heavily influenced by managers and leaders, within both a unit and the entire institution. It is notoriously difficult to change, as it can sometimes take years to permanently disrupt deeply embedded practices and to generate a new culture. When leadership provides an environment inhospitable to change or insufficient resources to implement those changes, devotion to traditional practices endures among staff. It is critical to preemptively identify and revise leadership and cultural barriers to QI initiatives.

Pitfall #7: Failure to Properly Use Automated Systems and the Electronic Medical Record

The electronic medical record (EMR) has been both a blessing and a curse for clinical practice, and its use in QI is no different. We have experienced both EMR extremes during an attempt to decrease the incidence of postoperative VTE. We developed a mandatory clinical decision support tool within the EMR that integrated the Caprini risk-assessment and prophylaxis system (Cassidy et al. 2014). "Hard stops" in the EMR require the selection of both risk level assignment and corresponding prophylaxis order options, eliminating the human behavior element of neglect. As a result, our VTE performance for General Surgery steadily moved from the worst decile (odds ratio, 3.02) in NSQIP to the best decile (odds ratio, 0.75) (Fig. 7.1). This success has promoted the diffusion of these automated VTE practices among the other surgery services at our institution. The application of the EMR to support clinical decision tools can be quite effective, especially when integrated into clinicians' workflow at precise moments of decision-making and of registering actionable recommendations (Kawamoto 2005).

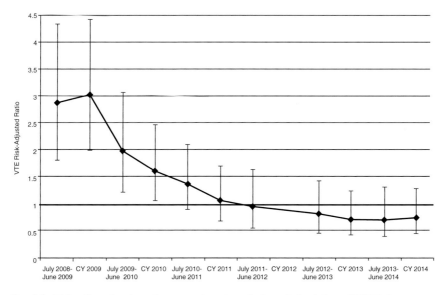

Fig. 7.1 Risk-adjusted ratios of venous thromboembolism derived from NSQIP data among General Surgery patients at Boston Medical Center, before and after final implementation of the Caprini program in February 2011

On the other hand, overreliance on the EMR can also be a pitfall. As an increasing number of best practice alerts inundate EMR workflow, they may become bothersome and less effective. Furthermore, software design is time consuming and requires resources that may not be readily available. Not every aspect of a project needs to be (or can be) electronically automated, and certain efforts may be better implemented with other strategies. In addition, the EMR can actually lead to technical errors that result in patient safety events. For example, when transitioning from one EMR system to another, the rebuilt Caprini system acquired a programming error that resulted in a peculiar subset of patients being prescribed a doubled dosage of VTE prophylaxis. A diligent clinician noticed an errant prescription and triggered an investigation and correction. When order options become automatic, providers may unintentionally abandon clinical reasoning, and errors of this nature could persist for extended intervals until being recognized.

Pitfall #8: Failure to Be Flexible and Adapt a Project Over Time

One of the biggest differences between QI and traditional research trials involves the ability to modify a protocol over time. A major pitfall in QI work is failing to revise or suspend a project when it is ineffective. To address the high rate of postoperative pulmonary complications revealed in initial NSQIP reports, we designed a bundled intervention of basic nursing and respiratory best practices, outlined by the acronym ICOUGH (Incentive spirometer, Coughing and deep breathing, Oral care, Understand/education, Get out of bed, and Head of bed elevation, all of which were embedded in standardized EMR order sets) (Cassidy et al. 2013). We observed an initial decrease in complication rates, but these rates increased once again as compliance with the recommendations declined and chronic habits returned. While this initiative, heavily dependent on changing behavioral practices, ultimately resulted in an overall decrease in the likelihood of pulmonary complications such as pneumonia, its progress has been charted in a saw-tooth pattern (Fig. 7.2), rather than in a smooth decline as seen with the automated Caprini system in Fig. 7.1. Causes of lapses included the loss of institutional support of personnel engaged in audits, data feedback, and patient education, the inability to quickly establish ICOUGH as the standard of care across various surgery specialties, misinterpretation of performance data distribution as confrontational rather than collegial, and loss of novelty over time. In fact, a nursing leader memorably proclaimed, "I thought ICOUGH is out this year, and patient satisfaction is in!" The constant redirection of priorities and support in any organization is perhaps the greatest threat to and pitfall of QI work.

The ICOUGH effort has required regular reinforcement, including redoubled education of patients and their families, improved data feedback to frontline staff, selection of local nurse champions, extended efforts on other surgery services and in the intensive care units, formal preoperative smoking cessation, and greater surveillance of patients at highest risk. We have realized that an acronym alone is insufficient to support long-term change and have instead fashioned a more com-

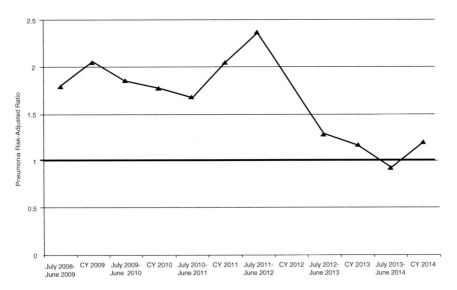

Fig. 7.2 Risk-adjusted ratios for pneumonia derived from NSQIP data among General Surgery patients at Boston Medical Center, before and after implementation of the ICOUGH program in August 2010

prehensive postoperative pulmonary program over time to buttress the original tenets of ICOUGH.

Another example of flexibility from the ICOUGH program resides in it having been originally designed exclusively for General Surgery patients. However, the ward nurses, educated about the pulmonary advantages promised by ICOUGH, questioned why they should deprive other patients of these best practices. In response, ICOUGH was uniformly delivered to all patients on those units. This experience exemplifies the value of listening to staff and being flexible. It also demonstrates that it can be taxing to discriminate among patients on a single unit.

There is no doubt that chance favors the prepared. As a result, one should not ignore the good fortune of unexpected support. For example, when we originally conceived both the ICOUGH and Caprini programs, it was a consultant's recommendation of a bowel resection protocol that provided the necessary dedication of information technology resources. We used that opportunity to create order sets that universally conveyed ICOUGH and Caprini elements for all patients on our service, along with other desired components of care related to bowel operations. While it is impossible to plan for such serendipity, it is important to seize upon support that may come from parallel projects. Graciously accept help and resources when offered.

Even a well-designed program should be periodically evaluated in order to allow opportunity to adapt to sustain desired practices. For example, education sessions and compliance audits are often planned only during a project's implementation, even though one can predict a regular turnover of frontline staff. The absence of a strategy for continued maintenance is a pitfall that can hinder even the most elegant QI projects from achieving prolonged change. Sustainability is frequently compromised when there is over-reliance on certain individuals or when assumptions are made that interventions will spontaneously diffuse and become standard practice (Dixon-Woods et al. 2012). Sustainability should not be an afterthought, and discussion about how to preserve QI changes should begin at an early stage.

Conclusion

Nearly all of the barriers and pitfalls presented above derive from personal experiences. Nevertheless, these moments have steeled us and have resulted in progressively more successful initiatives. At the start of this journey, the NSQIP odds ratio for postoperative complications in General Surgery at our institution was about 1.1; during recent years it has declined to 0.85–0.92. Keys to success include standardization when possible, risk assessment and risk-stratified care, standards that span multiple surgery services, persistent coordination and education of QI teams, and enhanced education of patients, families, and staff. In addition, we seek simplicity of efforts, automation to the extent possible, and problems with the greatest opportunity for improvement. Regular, constructive feedback is so important, especially when process measures can be matched to outcomes. Of course, the right personnel and leadership are critical in solidifying a commitment to quality as the essence of the organization's culture.

When disappointed by a QI lapse, we recall Thomas Edison's claim: "I have not failed. I've just found 10,000 ways that won't work". Surgical QI is difficult and often frustrating. It is easy to become pessimistic when a project does not proceed according to plan or when it is ineffective. However, it is imperative to persist, to regard failures as opportunities to learn, and to adapt and continuously improve the care of patients. In other words, don't give up! While there are innumerable potential QI pitfalls, we hope this chapter serves as a useful guide to avoid or at least circumnavigate frequently encountered impediments.

References

BMJ Quality improvement reports – BMJ Journals. 2015. http://qir.bmj.com/. Accessed 15 Dec 2015.

Bradley EH, Holmboe ES, Mattera JA, Roumanis SA, Radford MJ, Krumholz HM. Data feedback efforts in quality improvement: lessons learned from US hospitals. Qual Saf Health Care. 2004;13(1):26–31. doi:10.1136/qhc.13.1.26.

Cassidy MR, Rosenkranz P, McAneny D. Reducing postoperative venous thromboembolism complications with a standardized risk-stratified prophylaxis protocol and mobilization program. J Am Coll Surg. 2014;218(6):1095–104. doi:10.1016/j.jamcollsurg.2013.12.061.

Cassidy MR, Rosenkranz P, McCabe K, Rosen JE, McAneny D. I Cough: Reducing postoperative pulmonary complications with a multidisciplinary patient care program. JAMA Surg. 2013;148(8):740. doi:10.1001/jamasurg.2013.358.

Dixon-Woods M, McNicol S, Martin G. Ten challenges in improving quality in healthcare: lessons from the Health Foundation's programme evaluations and relevant literature. BMJ Qual Saf. 2012;21(10):876–84. doi:10.1136/bmjqs-2011-000760.

Gillies D. Hempelian and Kuhnian approaches in the philosophy of medicine: the Semmelweis case. Stud Hist Philos Sci Part C Stud Hist Philos Biol Biomed Sci. 2005;36(1):159–81. doi:10.1016/j.shpsc.2004.12.003.

Kawamoto K. Improving clinical practice using clinical decision support systems: a systematic review of trials to identify features critical to success. BMJ. 2005;330(7494):765. doi:10.1136/bmj.38398.500764.8F.

O'Neill SM. How do quality improvement interventions succeed? Archetypes of success and failure. Santa Monica: RAND Corporation. 2011. http://www.rand.org/pubs/rgs_dissertations/RGSD282.html.

Perla R, Reid A, Cohen S, Parry G. Health care reform and the trap of the "Iron Law." Health Affairs Blog. 2015. http://healthaffairs.org/blog/2015/04/22/health-care-reform-and-the-trap-of-the-iron-law/. Accessed 15 Dec 2015.

Pronovost PJ. Navigating adaptive challenges in quality improvement. BMJ Qual Saf. 2011;20(7):560–3. doi:10.1136/bmjqs-2011-000026.

Uberoi V, Calixte N, Coronel RV, Furlong JD, Orlando PR, Lerner BL. Reducing urinary catheter days. Nurs (Lond). 2013;43(1):16–20. doi:10.1097/01.NURSE.0000423971.46518.4d.

Urbach DR, Govindarajan A, Saskin R. Introduction of surgical safety checklists in Ontario, Canada. N Engl J Med. 2014;370(11):1029–38. doi:10.1016/j.jvs.2014.05.036.

Chapter 8
Conflict Resolution

Lawrence Tsen, Jo Shapiro, and Stanley Ashley

Abstract Conflicts occur frequently in the healthcare environment, and can stem from failures in communication, the presence of disruptive behaviors, and differences in values or priorities. A collaborative approach to conflict resolution, which focuses on an open, non-threatening exploration of issues and alternatives, creates optimal outcomes for interested parties. Conflict intensity can alter the participants' willingness to achieve a solution, and communication strategies should honor those emotions, while creating a neutral environment where dialogue can occur. Conflict management skills can be learned, and effectively employed for institutional and individual benefit.

> **Key Points**
> - Conflict occurs frequently within healthcare, and particularly in the operating room environment.
> - Conflict fosters decreased collaboration, employee satisfaction and patient safety, and can have significant institutional and individual implications.
> - The basic sources of conflict include failures in communication, the presence of disruptive behaviors, and differences in values or priorities.

L. Tsen
Center for Professionalism and Peer Support, Department of Anesthesiology, Perioperative and Pain Medicine, Brigham and Women's Hospital, Boston, MA, USA

Harvard Medical School, Boston, MA, USA

J. Shapiro
Center for Professionalism and Peer Support, Department of Surgery, Brigham and Women's Hospital, Boston, MA, USA

Harvard Medical School, Boston, MA, USA

S. Ashley (✉)
Harvard Medical School, Boston, MA, USA

Department of Surgery, Brigham and Women's Hospital, Boston, MA, USA
e-mail: SASHLEY@PARTNERS.ORG

© Springer International Publishing Switzerland 2017
R.R. Kelz, S.L. Wong (eds.), *Surgical Quality Improvement*,
Success in Academic Surgery, DOI 10.1007/978-3-319-23356-7_8

- Conflict evolves through different stages from participants not being fully aware of issues to overt manifestations of anger and stress.
- Participants' assertiveness and cooperativeness yield five distinct styles for responding to conflict: avoiding, accommodating, cooperating, compromising and collaborating. Collaborating produces the optimal results.
- Analyzing the source of conflict, understanding the positions, acknowledging possible and preferred solutions and creating a plan that assigns roles and tasks can improve conflict resolution.
- Conflict intensity, and their associated emotional states, can influence participants' willingness and ability to achieve a solution.
- The use of basic precepts during conflict resolution conversations can create a more open, communicative environment.
- Lasting solutions to conflict require participants to trust the intentions and promises of the other party.
- Conflict management skills can be learned and developed, and can be used to alter outcomes and relationships.

Introduction

Conflicts occur routinely in the healthcare environment. Your patient, armed with information obtained from the internet, insists that a different surgical approach would lead to a better outcome. The nurse refuses to draw the labs you ordered 6 hours ago because the requisition form was incomplete. The anesthesiologist delays your case until a cardiologist reviews what you perceive to be a normal electrocardiogram. Your surgical colleague jests that he contacted a malpractice attorney on your behalf regarding your complicated, just completed, operation.

Defined as a process in which perceived opposition between people or groups exists due to differences in interests, resources, beliefs, or values, (De Dreu and Gelfand 2008) conflict can lead to a number of outcomes. Personal or organizational growth can emerge from conflict, (Caudron 2000) particularly when the interaction is task oriented, and accomplished in a positive, trusting, environment (Tjosvold 2000).

However, conflict can also have dysfunctional, disruptive, or even destructive consequences, which can have significant implications to the involved individuals and institutions (Alper 2000). Alterations in productivity, work place or career satisfaction, job turnover and absenteeism, family well-being, and reputation in the medical (and legal) community can result (De Dreu 2010). Moreover, conflict can escalate in intensity, produce aggressive behavior, and lead into a spiral of unintended and unpredictable outcomes (Mikolic et al. 1997). Once promising surgical careers have ended due to poorly managed conflicts.

In observational studies of the surgical environment, an average of one to four conflicts occur among operating room teams during each operation (Booij 2007;

Saxton 2012). Within health care teams, conflicts have lead to reductions in communication, collaboration, and ultimately, patient satisfaction and safety (Joint Commission).

The reduction of conflict is therefore valuable to individuals as well as institutions; objective evaluations of the quality of communication and relationships, deemed relational coordination, can alter clinical outcomes. In 878 patients undergoing total hip and knee arthroplasty at nine independent hospitals, variation in relational coordination between health care providers has been associated with significant differences in satisfaction, postoperative pain and function, and even length of stay (Gittell et al. 2000). Consequently, understanding the sources and methods for managing conflict are paramount to a successful surgical career.

Sources and Stages of Conflict

Recognizing the principal source(s) of conflict can be helpful in diminishing or resolving a situation. Although the genesis of conflict may seem trivial (e.g., "He changed the radio station without asking...at a key point in the surgery!"), the underlying issues often involve essential differences in values, perspectives or priorities, failures in communication, or the presence of disruptive behaviors.

Values represent our personal beliefs of right or wrong. Reflected in how and why we make decisions, values are a core feature of our belief system. Although it is often difficult to articulate or even recognize individual values, it is difficult to compromise when our basic system of beliefs is challenged (Harolds and Wood 2006). Conflicts can also stem from differences in perspectives (e.g., lack of clarity of role or jurisdiction, interpretations of existing workload), priorities (e.g., efficiency of patient throughput), or personality attributes (e.g., limited emotional intelligence, introversion).

Communication failures can amplify these differences, particularly when inadequate, incorrect, or excessive information is provided (Table 8.1) (Saltman et al. 2006). Ongoing or unresolved communication failures or prior conflicts with you or individuals in a role identical to yours (e.g., "You surgical residents are all the same!") can lead to prejudiced initial viewpoints.

Finally, the work environment, including workload and stress, and organizational culture may engender conflicts between individuals or teams. Over time, dysfunctional experiences lead to adjusted behaviors that can negatively impact the

Table 8.1 Information patterns that lead to communication failures and conflict

Inadequate	Incorrect	Excessive
"Why won't you answer my emails and pages?" "Look, I don't have time to tell you how to do it...it's self-explanatory...just get it done"	"You gave me the results on the wrong patient" "You said to start the antibiotics *before* the sample was taken"	"Here are the 25 charts... the discharge note is likely in one of them"

Table 8.2 Stages of conflict

Conflict stage	Description	Example
Latent	Participants not yet aware	A necessary surgical instrument is missing from the kit opened for a case.
Perceived	Participants aware a conflict exists	After surgery has commenced, the scrub nurse mentions that the instrument is missing.
Felt	Participants feel stress and anxiety	The surgery cannot proceed without the instrument.
Manifest	Conflict is open and can be observed	Various participants blame others for the missing instrument. Tempers flare, supervisors are paged to the room, phone calls are made.
Aftermath	Conflict resolution or dissolution occurs	The needed surgical instrument is located, sterilized, and brought to the room. Appropriate steps are taken to minimize a reoccurrence.

relationships as well as the individuals involved (Song et al. 2000). Such behaviors, especially when emotionally charged, can become disruptive or destructive.

Conflict has been categorized into different stages (Table 8.2), which can be visualized as a bell shaped curve (Robbins and Judge 2014). When participant(s) first perceive conflict, resolution can be sought. However, conflicts typically build until a triggering event elicits the manifest stage during which enhanced discomfort leads to altered behavior and visible or obvious conflict (e.g., passive aggressive behavior, disruptive actions or activities, etc.).

Manifestations of conflict are often best mitigated if addressed earlier; however, the duration and movement through conflict stages is dependent on a number of variables. The ramifications of a missing surgical instrument, for example, would differ if an easily substitutable instrument was already present on the surgical tray.

Responses to Conflict

Although some organizations have processes to assist conflict management, the participants involved determine the initial, and often ongoing, actions and responses.

A number of variables, including personality, roles, presence of power or hierarchy, rewards, attitudes, perceptions, ethnicity, and gender, can influence responses to conflict. Psychosocial studies, especially those based on the Thomas Killman Conflict Mode Instrument, have validated the presence of five distinct styles in responding to conflict; the styles can be visualized on a matrix using two axes of assertiveness and cooperativeness (Thomas 1992; Fig. 8.1).

The five styles are avoiding, accommodating, competing, collaborating, and compromising. Avoiding, which is the most frequent response to conflict, is both unassertive and uncooperative; it allows the conflict to continue and possibly flourish. By contrast, collaborating is both assertive and cooperative, and represents a direct attempt to resolve the conflict; it is considered to be the optimal style. The

High

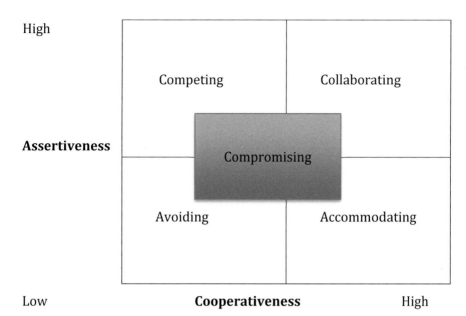

Assertiveness

Low   **Cooperativeness**   High

Fig. 8.1 Conflict mode instrument. The four basic "modes" or styles of responding to conflict based on the elements of assertiveness or cooperativeness. The "compromising" style has features of two or more styles, but is not the most effective. The "collaborating" style yields the optimal outcomes for participants

collaborating style requires an open, non-threatening discussion of issues, an imaginative exploration of alternatives, and honesty and commitment; the style can merge insights from people on different "sides" of a problem, and result in commitment to the solution. This style is not to be confused with compromising, which has each interested party give up or trade desired elements; resulting solutions can often lead to agreements where no one is satisfied.

As individuals gain experience or leadership positions, there is a tendency to use more assertive, less cooperative methods (i.e., competing). Novice or less experienced individuals (e.g., intern) have a tendency to engage in less assertive, more cooperative methods (i.e., accommodating) (Slabbert 2004). Hierarchical organizations, such as surgical or medical environments, tend to embrace less cooperative methods at higher levels, reflecting the dominance-subservience patterns that often exist. However, individuals should still strive to be both assertive and cooperative (i.e., collaborative) to improve conflict resolution success.

A second model of conflict resolution defines negotiating styles in accordance with the extent to which the negotiator attempts to satisfy their own interests and consider the other party's interests (Rahim 1995). These dimensions can be visualized on two axes yielding four pure categories (Fig. 8.2), with the fifth category "compromising" being a moderate position encompassing interests of self and others. Forcing is distinguished into direct fighting (i.e., uses result-oriented mechanisms such as threats, and physical or verbal violence) and indirect fighting (i.e., controls

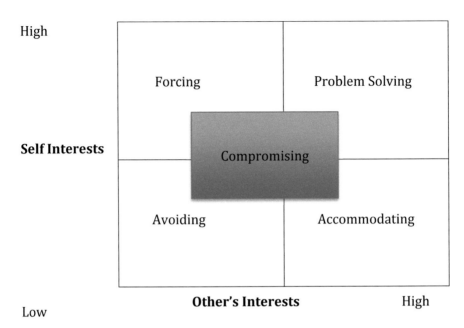

High

Self Interests

Forcing

Problem Solving

Compromising

Avoiding

Accommodating

Low

Other's Interests   High

Fig. 8.2 Conflict mode instrument based on interests. The four basic "modes" or styles of responding to conflict based on elements of self- or other's- interests. The "compromising" style has features of two or more styles, but is not the most effective. The problem solving style yields the
optimal outcomes for participants

the process or resists considering the adversary's issues) (Van de Vliert 1994). Not
surprisingly, problem solving is the most successful option, as it enables both parties to consider a greater number of positions and counter-positions and places
greater effort into satisfying underlying needs (Putnam and Wilson 1989) to reach a
mutually satisfactory agreement (Medina and Benitez).

Management of Conflict

Conflict should be addressed, particularly when the possibility of real or potential
injury exists (e.g., a participant's psychological health or a patient's outcome) or a
high likelihood of affecting subsequent behavior is present. Although soliciting a
third party to resolve conflict has some appeal, such an approach is not realistic for
many common issues; moreover, organizations, as well as individuals not person-
ally involved, can have difficulties in managing conflict constructively and resulting
delays can diminish memory of important provoking or contributing elements
(Slabbert 2004). As importantly, conflict management skills are essential to achieving personal growth and development, and improving the workplace environment.

Initiating a conversation to resolve conflict requires preparation, including analyzing the source(s) and intensity of the conflict, understanding the positions

(including yours), acknowledging the possible and preferred solutions, and creating a plan that assigns roles and tasks.

Runde and Flanagan (2010) describe five levels of conflict intensity between two or more participants with different perspectives (Table 8.3). The intensity of the situation, with its associated emotional states, can influence the participants' willingness to approach and achieve a solution. Addressing conflict should ideally occur when the acute sensations of anger, frustration or hurt have somewhat dissipated, but the triggering or situational factors can still be recalled. Mitigating emotional states can lead to calmer and clearer discussions; tension reduction has been achieved by creating awareness of behaviors that provoke emotional responses and reframing perspectives from an alternative, generally more positive viewpoint.

In the presence of conflict escalation, certain behaviors, mostly related to accommodation, can assist in diffusing tension. "Influence tactics" include acknowledging their principle concerns, convincing the other individual(s) that your opinion of them is positive, which facilitates relations and increase trust (Wayne 1997), and making public concessions, which obliges the other party to consider or make concessions as well (Osgood 1962). For example, if a patient is vocally aggressive and agitated with clinic schedule delays in the waiting room, having someone approach them, agree that the clinic has not been punctual, acknowledge the value of their time, and offer the option of their going for a walk and receiving a text message at the appropriate time, will likely benefit all parties involved. Such accommodations can then facilitate a fuller, later conversation to potentially evaluate root causes for the conflict and diminish future similar encounters.

The use of basic precepts and mindsets can foster a more open, sharing environment for communication to occur (Table 8.4). As negotiations begin, the quality of the process and outcome depend on the frequency, as well as the distribution, of a given strategy; constructive resolutions most often occur when a negotiator is firm and resilient in the early phases, but flexible and creative in later stages (Medina and Benitez 2011). Conversely, ineffective influence tactics are often based on the use of demonstrable force, including launching personal attacks and trivializing the other party's issue; adopting soft styles of avoidance and servility are also not effective in creating lasting solutions (Munduate et al. 1999). Finally, being firm and inflexible late in the negotiations process often leads to negotiation failure.

Table 8.3 Conflict intensity levels

Intensity level	Term	Description
1	Difference	Participants understand and are comfortable with the other's viewpoint
2	Misunderstanding	Participants understand the situation differently
3	Disagreement	Participants understand, yet are uncomfortable, with viewing the situation differently
4	Discord	Participants may have a specific conflict resolved, but have an impaired relationship
5	Polarization	Participants have intense negative behaviors and feelings towards a relationship

Table 8.4 Tips for engaging a conflict resolution conversation

Element	Value
Moving to a neutral space	Removes the interaction away from colleagues or patients, where "losing face" or "allies jumping in" can complicate considerations.
Sharing the impact	Identifies how the comment, behavior or action alters the environment as well as your (and others) feelings.
Inviting their perspectives	Allows the other individual(s) an opportunity to share reasons or events provoking their behavior(s).
Altering your internal voice	Diminishes attacking their comments or explanations or labeling the individual(s) or issues as non-alterable.
Mirroring behaviors	Allows the other party greater comfort during the conversation e.g., leaning back or taking a pause may indicate a need to reflect; this is likely not the optimal time to take a more aggressive tact.
Listening and paraphrasing	Exemplifies that the issues being shared are acknowledged and understood.

Understanding the differences inherent to the conflict include evaluating the background factual basis and data, anticipating the contrasting viewpoint's arguments, achieving clarity on what defines desirable and undesirable outcomes, and considering reasonable concessions. The greatest potential for a workable solution exists when both parties understand the value of a long-term relationship and achieve an outcome that satisfies or exceeds their anticipated gain. An optimal outcome is one that encompasses mutual understanding and benefit; ideally, it is a solution whereby additional benefits for one party cannot be achieved without reducing those for the other party.

In seeking a lasting solution, participants must believe that they will be respected and treated fairly. The participants must trust in the intentions of the other party, with an expectation that confidentiality for disclosed information will be maintained, and promises tendered will be honored. Such a solution has roles and tasks that each party fulfills as an indicator of actively incorporating the agreement as well as strengthening the relationship.

Following conflict, further relationship building acknowledges the need for acknowledging a mutual purpose or goal, identifying and solving problems, and seeking opportunities for ongoing communication to resolve misunderstandings or irritations to the relationship.

Conclusion

Conflicts occur frequently in the healthcare environment, and can stem from failures in communication, the presence of disruptive behaviors, and differences in values or priorities. A collaborative approach to conflict resolution, which focuses on an open, non-threatening exploration of issues and alternatives, creates optimal outcomes for interested parties. Conflict intensity can alter the participants' willingness to achieve a solution, and communication strategies should honor those emotions, while creating a neutral environment where dialogue can occur. Conflict management skills can be learned, and effectively employed for institutional and individual benefit.

References

Alper S. Conflict management, efficacy and performance in organizational teams. Pers Psychol. 2000;53:625–42.

Booij LH. Conflicts in the operating theatre. Curr Opin Anaesthesiol. 2007;20(2):152–6.

Caudron S. Keeping team conflict alive: conflict can be a good thing. Public Manage. 2000;82:5–9.

De Dreu CKW. Social conflict: the emergence and consequences of struggle and negotiation. In: Fiske ST, Gilbert DT, Lindzey G, editors. Handbook of social psychology. 5th ed. New York: Wiley; 2010. p. 983–1023.

De Dreu CKW, Gelfand MJ. The psychology of conflict and conflict management in organizations. New York: Lawrence Erlbaum Associates Taylor & Francis Group; 2008.

Gittell JH, et al. Impact of relational coordination on quality of care, postoperative pain and functioning, and length of stay: a nine-hospital study of surgical patients. Med Care. 2000;38(8):807–19.

Harolds J, Wood BP. Conflict management and resolution. J Am Coll Radiol. 2006;3(3):200–6.

Medina FJ, Benitez M. Effective behaviors to de-escalate organizational conflicts in the process of escalation. Span J Psychol. 2011;14(2):789–97.

Mikolic JM, et al. Escalation in response to persistent annoyance: groups versus individuals and gender effects. J Pers Soc Psychol. 1997;72(1):151–63.

Munduate L, et al. Patterns of styles in conflict management and effectiveness. Int J Confl Manage. 1999;10:5–24.

Osgood CE. An alternative to war or surrender. Urbana: University of Illinois Press; 1962.

Putnam LL, Wilson SR. Argumentation and bargaining strategies as discriminators of integrative outcomes. In M. A. Rahim (Ed.), Managing conflict: An interdisciplinary approach. New York, NY: Praeger. 1989. p. 121–41.

Rahim MA, Magner NR. Confirmatory factor analysis of the styles of handling interpersonal conflict: first-order factor model and its invariance across groups. J Appl Psychol. 1995;80(1):122–32.

Robbins SP, Judge TA. Organizational behavior. Upper Saddle River: Prentice Hall; 2014.

Runde C, Flanagan T. Developing you conflict competence: a hands-on guide for leaders, managers, facilitators, and teams. San Francisco: Jossey-Bass; 2010.

Saltman DC, et al. Conflict management: a primer for doctors in training. Postgrad Med J. 2006;82(963):9–12.

Saxton R. Communication skills training to address disruptive physician behavior. AORN J. 2012;95(5):602–11.

Slabbert AD. Conflict management styles in traditional organisations. Soc Sci J. 2004;41(1):83–92.

Song XM, et al. Antecedents and consequences of marketing managers' conflict-handling behaviors. J Mark. 2000;64:50–66.

Thomas, Kenneth W. Conflict and conflict management: reflections and update. J Organ Behav 1992;(13):265–74.

Tjosvold D. Learning to manage conflict: getting people to work together productively. New York: Lexington Books; 2000.

van de Vliert E1, Euwema MC. Agreeableness and activeness as components of conflict behaviors. J Pers Soc Psychol. 1994;66(4):674–87.

Wayne SJ, Liden RC, Graf IK, Ferris GR. The role of upward influence tactics in human resource decisions. Personnel Psychology. 1997;50:979–1006.

Chapter 9
Teaching Quality Improvement

Morgan M. Sellers, Sandra L. Wong, and Rachel R. Kelz

Abstract As issues of patient safety and quality assurance have come to the fore-front of national discussions regarding medical care in the past two decades, there has been a simultaneous recognition that these topics must be addressed in medical education. The importance of developing expertise in teaching quality improvement (QI) is twofold: trainees are (1) the "front-line" providers in many healthcare institutions where their awareness and positive involvement in QI is crucial to the success of robust quality initiatives, and (2) the future practitioners who will shape the next generation of quality work and face issues of quality and safety in daily practice.

Introduction

As issues of patient safety and quality assurance have come to the forefront of national discussions regarding medical care in the past two decades, there has been a simultaneous recognition that these topics must be addressed in medical education. The importance of developing expertise in teaching quality improvement (QI) is twofold: trainees are (1) the "front-line" providers in many healthcare institutions where their awareness and positive involvement in QI is crucial to the success of robust quality initiatives, and (2) the future practitioners who will shape the next generation of quality work and face issues of quality and safety in daily practice.

There is a pressing need to implement quality improvement education in surgical training. As measures of quality and patient safety (PS) have been adopted and followed by various governmental and other organizing bodies, these topics have been

M.M. Sellers, MD (✉)
Department of Surgery, Icahn School of Medicine at Mount Sinai, New York, NY, USA
e-mail: morgan.sellers@gmail.com

S.L. Wong, MD, MS
The Geisel School of Medicine at Dartmouth, Hanover, NH, USA
e-mail: Sandra.L.Wong@dartmouth.edu

R.R. Kelz, MD, MSCE
Perelman School of Medicine, University of Pennsylvania, Philadelphia, PA, USA

© Springer International Publishing Switzerland 2017   85
R.R. Kelz, S.L. Wong (eds.), *Surgical Quality Improvement*,
Success in Academic Surgery, DOI 10.1007/978-3-319-23356-7_9

included in the defined goals of medical education. There is now a growing body of literature regarding mechanisms for including quality improvement and patient safety in both undergraduate and graduate medical education. However there is variation in adoption and dissemination and a defined knowledge gap in best practices for surgical educators. The goal of this chapter is to outline the current developing efforts to teach QI in surgery, primarily at the graduate medical education (GME) level, as well as to highlight best practices and lay out guidelines for the ongoing development of programs.

Background

Over the past two decades, issues of safety and quality have risen to the forefront of national discussions regarding healthcare, driven by increasing awareness of the role of medical errors in patient mortality (Kohn et al. 1999; Makary and Daniel 2016) and efforts to understand and control the rising costs of healthcare. In this context, there has been a growing mandate to include these topics in medical training. Perhaps the most influential was the development of the six core competencies by the Accreditation Council for Graduate Medical Education (ACGME) in 1999. These comprise medical knowledge, patient care, communication, professionalism, systems based practice (SBP), and practice based learning and improvement (PBLI). While various aspects of quality improvement and patient safety map onto all six of the ACGME core competencies, SBP and PBLI encompass many of the specific topics and skills that were previously not typically included in residency education, and provide a clear directive to include these concepts in residency education.

Following the formulation of these required areas of medical training, there was a large amount of experimentation by graduate medical education programs in ways to include SBP and PBLI (and by extension QI/PS) in their curricula. In 2005, a national consensus conference on patient safety education in surgery was jointly sponsored by the American College of Surgeons (ACS) and the Association for Surgical Education (ASE), and attended by leaders of the ACGME and the American Board of Medical Specialties (ABM) as well as representatives from the Surgical Residency Review Committees, American Board of Surgery, American Surgical Association, and Association of Program Directors in Surgery, as well as surgical residents. The recommendations and guidelines from that conference mapped patient safety topics to each of the six ACGME competencies and offered suggestions on specific ways to introduce each into the resident curriculum. The consensus statement specifically recommended developing a "standardized introductory course on patient safety", the development of "longitudinal educational programs" in patient safety, and linking patient safety education with other educational activities (Sachdeva et al. 2007).

A number of studies have since reviewed and analyzed published reports of QI/PS curricula in different medical specialties. The first review, published in 2007, identified seven studies targeting residents (Boonyasai et al. 2007). Subsequent reviews in 2010 and 2016 identified 27 and 44 studies targeting residents respectively (Wong et al. 2010; Starr et al. 2016). A 2014 review specifically focused on quality improvement curricula targeted to surgical fields found 31 articles describing GME curricula, with only six specific to surgery (Medbery et al. 2014).

Despite the clear growth in published examples, many of the issues identified in the first review remain true, and are instructive for institutions looking to develop their own curricula: most curricula describe isolated QI projects with minimal interdisciplinary interaction, and are challenged by lack of experienced teachers or coaches. Additionally, few reports have described projects with rigorously measured patient or care outcomes, instead focusing on knowledge acquisition or changes in learner attitudes.

Educational Framework

In the setting of surgical education, quality improvement must be approached both as a knowledge set as well as a driving culture. As the curricular reviews above point out, the best educational approach will not be a solitary isolated curriculum but rather an integration of QI principles, attitudes, and skills throughout training. A multipronged approach is necessary to include all these components. The challenge for each institution is to find the right combination of resources (e.g., stand-alone curricula, hands-on projects, and integration into existing QI efforts).

Isolating the discussion or teaching of QI skills from hands-on patient care activities can result in trainees seeing QI as an isolated "barrier" to care as opposed to an integral constructive necessary part. Therefore, in teaching QI, it is important to consider both the defined curricula used to teach specific skills, but also the "hidden curricula" that trainees are exposed to. It is important to note that there is no unified consensus on what comprise the key components of quality improvement and patient safety (Moran et al. 2016). It is useful to think about QI education as being constructed of a few different components, each of which must be addressed in order to provide trainees with the necessary skills to succeed. Here, we have chosen to break down methods of teaching knowledge, skills, and attitudes as three separate components that should each be addressed.

Foundational Knowledge and Didactics

The most straightforward of these components to address is the transmission of knowledge, typically in the form of didactics. Table 9.1 lists some of the more commonly listed topics covered in reported curricula, divided into different domains. These include foundational concepts in patient safety and quality improvement, as well as defined techniques in each of these fields such as Lean Six Sigma (a process improvement methodology that was developed in industrial engineering and has

Table 9.1 Key didactic components of QI curricula (foundational knowledge)

Domain	Selected topics
Basics of patient safety	Scope and impact of medical errors
	Types of error (e.g., Swiss cheese model)
	Safety culture
	Importance of near misses
	Root cause analysis
Basics of quality improvement	Continuous quality improvement techniques (e.g., PDSA cycle)
	Process improvement techniques (e.g., Lean Six Sigma)
	Outcomes measurement
Health care systems and structures	Overview of structure of US healthcare system
	Payments and incentives
Implementation science	Understanding complex systems
	Barriers to change
	Human factors
Leadership, teamwork, and communication	Principles of teamwork
	Components of successful teams
	Importance of handoffs
	Communication strategies following adverse events

been widely adopted at the institutional level in healthcare). Almost all described curricula include topics covering the basics of QI and PS. Depending on the intended extent and scope, related domains such as health care systems, implementation science, leadership, and communication are often also covered. There are a number of stand-alone resources that have been extensively developed that can provide a useful framework.

In 2008, the independent not-for-profit organization Institute for Healthcare Improvement (IHI) started a virtual "Open School" comprised of online modules and courses (including video and slideshows) covering a wide range of topics in patient safety and quality improvement as well as related domains such as communication and leadership (Institute for Healthcare Improvement 2016). IHI itself also provides a framework for the establishment of local chapters housed at health professions schools or hospitals around the globe. A number of the published QI curricula have used IHI Open School modules as a basis for self-paced learning that is then supplemented by group lectures or activities. Given the widespread adoption of the IHI Open School modules and robust methodology behind their development, this is a practical and easily accessible way for training programs to access high-quality basic didactics (O'Heron and Jarman 2014), however the modules are not specific to surgery.

The Quality In-Training Initiative, a collaborative of training programs participating in the American College of Surgeons National Surgical Quality Improvement Program, developed and released a surgery-specific QI curriculum in 2014 entitled "Practical QI", designed to introduce the key concepts of QI and guide surgical residents through the development and implementation of a basic QI project (Ko et al. 2014). Lesson plans linked to the Practical QI materials are published on the Surgical Council on Resident Education (SCORE) platform (SCORE 2016).

In contrast to a designated separate QI curriculum, individual institutions have developed their own QI curricula (Waits et al. 2014; O'Connor et al. 2010; Canal et al. 2007; Sellers et al. 2013a), or have published their experiences attempting to integrate QI topics into existing didactic structures, such as journal clubs (Lee et al. 2006) and bedside rounds. There have been few systematic or rigorous descriptions of these efforts, and we believe the best approach for each institution likely includes a combination of existing didactics (such as SCORE modules or IHI) and use of local expertise in QI.

Experiential Learning: Hands-On QI

The second component of QI education consists of the development of hands-on skills. A variety of projects and structures have been described at the undergraduate and graduate medical education levels and in a variety of different clinical fields. Many of the curricula included in the large reviews described above include these kinds of activities. In the surgical education literature, the most commonly described QI projects involves a small group of residents selecting a topic of interest and developing a quality intervention. These types of projects are now becoming a mainstay of poster and podium presentations at all levels of research conferences, ranging from the institutional to the national. On face value there is obvious benefit to trainees in participating in such projects, but as the reviews above note, few studies have been designed to clearly test the impact of participation either on trainees or on patient outcomes. This is in part a result of the time scale of most of the published studies, which often describe only the initial implementation or first 1–2 years of a given program, which does not give enough time to measure and report the effects of such curricula on the participants themselves, or to accurately measure the long term effects of QI projects that come out of these curricula.

A similar challenge relates to whether a project is conceived as a one-time initiative or as an ongoing effort; if the goal is to develop the latter (preferred from an institutional and outcomes perspective given limited resources for support of large scale implementation of many projects), then mechanisms to handoff a project to the next set of trainees must also be included in the overall project design (Patow et al. 2009). Finally, lack of qualified faculty to support and mentor trainees throughout a QI project is an ongoing challenge that is starting to be addressed with the development of faculty-specific curricula (Rodrigue et al. 2013; Myers and Nash 2014; Hull et al. 2015; Rao et al. 2016).

A variety of alternate types of experiential learning in QI have been described in other training disciplines that are worth noting as they may be applicable to an individual institutional setting. These include the development of a robust multispecialty housestaff counsel (Fleischut et al. 2012; Dixon et al. 2013), and participation in root-cause-analysis or clinical quality review activities (Ramanathan et al. 2015; Strayer et al. 2014).

Of particular importance to surgical departments is the role of morbidity and mortality conferences in trainee and departmental-wide QI activities. The reporting of cases can itself be seen as a QI activity at the trainee level, and has been studied (Hutter et al. 2006; Falcone et al. 2012), showing that overall complications are dramatically underreported, although serious complications are better reported. A number of studies have documented efforts to alter the structure or focus of M&M conferences to better highlight educational value, or to specifically focus on systems issues that can be more directly tied to principles of QI/PS (Kim et al. 2010).

An emerging focus in surgery is the analysis of patient process or outcome measures with more frequent occurrence rates than those typically discussed at the M&M level, such as timely use of correct antibiotics, rates of surgical site infections, or readmissions. This has been prompted by increasing ties of reimbursement to these measures. The ACS NSQIP QITI group has spearheaded the effort to introduce this skill at the trainee level, seeing this as a ripe opportunity for introducing residents to the types of data that are currently collected and will play increasingly important roles throughout their careers, as well as serving as a link between developing QI skills and ongoing patient care activities (Sellers et al. 2013b).

QI Culture and Attitudes

The third necessary component of QI education is the incorporation of the principles of implementation science into the overall environment and attitudes of the individual trainee and the institutional setting. There is a long history of self-reflection and data-driven improvement in surgery, dating to Ernest Codman's "end results" database, but more recent efforts to introduce systematic quality and safety measures into surgical environments have often faced resistance and had unforeseen consequences. Unfortunately, this has the tendency to set up a false conflict between patient care and patient safety.

Ways to address this at an organizational level are beyond the scope of this chapter, but it is clear that in training institutions, positive engagement of trainees is crucial to the success of both quality/safety efforts in some of our largest hospitals and healthcare systems, as well as to the future sustainability of these efforts in healthcare. The "hands-on" mechanisms for teaching QI skills that are described in the previous section can be key components of this if they are intentionally integrated into existing QI/PS efforts. These include long-term QI projects, participation in QI housestaff quality councils, and M&M conferences or case reviews.

One key component of organizational safety culture that has too rarely been incorporated into trainee-directed QI curricula is the importance of interdisciplinary coordination. In a healthcare system that has adopted and embraced a culture of safety, all members of the team must participate in QI activities, including physicians, staff, nurses, and other stakeholders. Many quality and safety challenges come at the interface of work between these different professionals, and can only be addressed as a team and by taking existing culture into consideration (Starr et al. 2016).

One key opportunity to integrate trainees into ongoing institutional efforts in QI/PS are staff team-based training requirements that often (unintentionally) exclude trainees. Arguably the most widespread of these is TeamSTEPPS, which was developed by the US Department of Defense and the Agency for Healthcare Research and Quality as a self-contained training module focusing on teamwork to improve healthcare quality, safety, and efficiency (King et al. 2008). A recent study looking at specific knowledge and attitude measurements after department-wide training in TeamSTEPPS in an academic emergency department (including residents), showed significant improvement in both (Lisbon et al. 2016).

Simulation

Simulation provides another unique opportunity in surgical training programs that can cross over between the three educational components listed above. The use of simulation in technical surgical education continues to expand and there is increasing knowledge and expertise in how to design modules that become useful adjuncts and preparations for in vivo surgical learning. Development in this realm has been pushed by concerns of patient safety and increasing supervision during technical procedures. Within the correct framework, technical simulation work can also function as a form of conscious self-improvement that trainees can recognize as a form of PBLI (Paige et al. 2015).

However, the role of simulation in non-technical skills is still evolving. Some key work has come out of high fidelity trainers such as the "SimMan" used in mock codes. Other areas, such as the management of other postop complications, are still being developed (Nicksa et al. 2015; Miyasaka et al. 2015; Arora et al. 2015; Dedy et al. 2013). The American College of Surgeons/Association of Program Directors in Surgery developed a comprehensive simulation curriculum for nontechnical skills, which includes such modules as managing postoperative hypotension, preoperative briefing, and intraoperative troubleshooting (phase III of the ACS/APDS skills curriculum), but adoption and implementation in training programs has been very slow (Hull et al. 2015). It is important to recognize that the use of simulation itself does not automatically contribute positively to a culture of safety, but rather can be an important component when it is properly integrated with other programs and includes appropriate coaching in self-reflection and self-improvement.

Assessment

As GME has moved towards an outcomes driven climate, assessment is becoming a crucial part of any educational intervention. The role of assessment in QI education is often discussed, but clear mechanisms for measuring trainees' competency have not yet been developed. Unfortunately, assessment has not typically been included in curricula or experiential learning. Of the three domains discussed above (knowledge, skills, and attitude), there are published tools for two these (knowledge and attitude).

The Quality Improvement Knowledge Application Tool (QIKAT), was first developed and described in 2003 (Ogrinc et al. 2004). It consists of three pretest and three posttest questions in which examinees are asked to respond to written scenarios describing quality or safety issues. Scores are graded subjectively. While it has not been formally validated, it has been shown to be able to distinguish groups of individuals with PBLI training and those without, and has now been used in a number of published studies as a way to measure change in individual knowledge on QI topics.

The second tool that is commonly used is the AHRQ patient safety culture survey, developed in 2004, a validated and free tool which measures 12 dimensions of patient safety culture such as communication openness, overall perceptions of safety, and teamwork within and across hospital units. Of note, this is a measurement of an organization's culture, not that of an individual participant.

As of yet, there is no widely used validated tool for measuring the ability of trainees to apply QI skills, highlighting the need for further development of multi-modal methods of both teaching and evaluation. The development of such a tool, along with further delineation of uniform curricular and skill-focused competencies for trainees should continue to be a priority for surgical educators.

Conclusion

The development of best-practices and robust methods for teaching QI and PS is ongoing. An increased appreciation for the importance of this topic is evolving, and, over the previous decade, a tremendous amount of groundwork has been performed, preparing surgical training programs to be receptive to these activities, and laying the foundation for the introduction of more rigorous curricula and activities. Innovative educational techniques and a global education of the surgical leadership on QI are critical to the advancement of the field. It is crucial that all three components of QI education be addressed (knowledge, skills, and attitudes) to prevent QI being seen as an isolated topic rather than an integrated and central component to future practice.

References

Arora S, Hull L, Fitzpatrick M, Sevdalis N, Birnbach DJ. Crisis management on surgical wards: a simulation-based approach to enhancing technical, teamwork, and patient interaction skills. Ann Surg. 2015;261(5):888–93.

Boonyasai RT, Windish DM, Chakraborti C, Feldman LS, Rubin HR, Bass EB. Effectiveness of teaching quality improvement to clinicians: a systematic review. JAMA. 2007;298(9):1023–37.

Canal DF, Torbeck L, Djuricich AM. Practice-based learning and improvement. Arch Surg. 2007;142(5):479–82.

Dedy NJ, Bonrath EM, Zevin B, Grantcharov TP. Teaching nontechnical skills in surgical residency: a systematic review of current approaches and outcomes. Surgery. 2013;154(5):1000–8.

Dixon JL, Papaconstantinou HT, Erwin 3rd JP, McAllister RK, Berry T, Wehbe-Janek H. House staff quality council: One Institution's experience to integrate resident involvement in patient care improvement initiatives. Ochsner J. 2013;13(3):394 9.

Falcone JL, Lee KK, Billiar TR, Hamad GG. Practice-based learning and improvement: a two-year experience with the reporting of morbidity and mortality cases by general surgery residents. J Surg Educ. 2012;69(3):385–92.

Fleischut PM, Faggiani SL, Evans AS, Brenner S, Liebowitz RS, Forese L, et al. 2011 John M. Eisenberg Patient Safety and Quality Awards. The effect of a novel housestaff quality council on quality and patient safety. Innovation in patient safety and quality at the local level. Jt Comm J Qual Patient Saf. 2012;38(7):311–7.

Hull L, Arora S, Stefanidis D, Sevdalis N. Facilitating the implementation of the American College of Surgeons/Association of Program Directors in surgery phase III skills curriculum: training faculty in the assessment of team skills. Am J Surg. 2015;210(5):933,41.e2.

Hutter MM, Rowell KS, Devaney LA, Sokal SM, Warshaw AL, Abbott WM, et al. Identification of surgical complications and deaths: an assessment of the traditional surgical morbidity and mortality conference compared with the American College of Surgeons-National Surgical Quality Improvement Program. J Am Coll Surg. 2006;203(5):618–24.

Institute for Healthcare Improvement: overview [Internet]. Institute for healthcare improvement; c2016 [cited 2016 Jun 20]. Available from: http://www.ihi.org/education/ihiopenschool/overview/Pages/default.aspx.

Kim MJ, Fleming FJ, Peters JH, Salloum RM, Monson JR, Eghbali ME. Improvement in educational effectiveness of morbidity and mortality conferences with structured presentation and analysis of complications. J Surg Educ. 2010;67(6):400–5.

King H, Battles J, Baker D. TeamSTEPPS™: team strategies and tools to enhance performance and patient safety. In: Henriksen K, Battles JB, Keyes MA, editors. Advances in patient safety: new directions and alternative approaches, Performance and tools, vol. 3. Rockville: Agency for Healthcare Research and Quality (US); 2008.

Ko CY, Kelz RR, editors. Practical QI: the basics of quality improvement (the quality in-training initiative: an ACS NSQIP collaborative). Chicago: American College of Surgeons; 2014.

Kohn L, Corrigan J, Donaldson M, editors. To err is human: building a safer health system. Washington DC: National Academies Press; 1999.

Lee AG, Boldt HC, Golnik KC, Arnold AC, Oetting TA, Beaver HA, et al. Structured journal club as a tool to teach and assess resident competence in practice-based learning and improvement. Ophthalmology. 2006;113(3):497–500.

Lisbon D, Allin D, Cleek C, Roop L, Brimacombe M, Downes C, et al. Improved knowledge, attitudes, and behaviors after implementation of TeamSTEPPS training in an academic emergency department: a pilot report. Am J Med Qual. 2016;31(1):86–90.

Makary MA, Daniel M. Medical error-the third leading cause of death in the US. BMJ. 2016;353:i2139.

Medbery RL, Sellers MM, Ko CY, Kelz RR. The unmet need for a national surgical quality improvement curriculum: a systematic review. J Surg Educ. 2014;71(4):613–31.

Miyasaka KW, Martin ND, Pascual JL, Buchholz J, Aggarwal R. A simulation curriculum for management of trauma and surgical critical care patients. J Surg Educ. 2015;72(5):803–10.

Moran KM, Harris IB, Valenta AL. Competencies for patient safety and quality improvement: a synthesis of recommendations in influential position papers. Jt Comm J Qual Patient Saf. 2016;42(4):162–9.

Myers JS, Nash DB. Graduate medical education's new focus on resident engagement in quality and safety: will it transform the culture of teaching hospitals? Acad Med. 2014;89(10):1328–30.

Nicksa GA, Anderson C, Fidler R, Stewart L. Innovative approach using interprofessional simu-
    lation to educate surgical residents in technical and nontechnical skills in high-risk clinical
    scenarios. JAMA Surg. 2015;150(3):201–7.
O'Connor ES, Mahvi DM, Foley EF, Lund D, McDonald R. Developing a practice-based learn-
    ing and improvement curriculum for an academic general surgery residency. J Am Coll Surg.
    2010;210(4):411–7.
O'Heron CT, Jarman BT. A strategic approach to quality improvement and patient safety education
    and resident integration in a general surgery residency. J Surg Educ. 2014;71(1):18–20.
Ogrinc G, Headrick LA, Morrison LJ, Foster T. Teaching and assessing resident competence in
    practice-based learning and improvement. J Gen Intern Med. 2004;19(5 Pt 2):496–500.
Paige JT, Yu Q, Hunt JP, Marr AB, Stuke LE. Thinking it through: mental rehearsal and perfor-
    mance on 2 types of laparoscopic cholecystectomy simulators. J Surg Educ. 2015;72(4):740–8.
Patow CA, Karpovich K, Riesenberg LA, Jaeger J, Rosenfeld JC, Wittenbreer M, et al. Residents'
    engagement in quality improvement: a systematic review of the literature. Acad Med.
    2009;84(12):1757–64.
Ramanathan R, Duane TM, Kaplan BJ, Farquhar D, Kasirajan V, Ferrada P. Using a root cause
    analysis curriculum for practice-based learning and improvement in general surgery residency.
    J Surg Educ. 2015;72(6):e286–93.
Rao SK, Carballo V, Cummings BM, Millham F, Jacobson JO. Developing an Interdisciplinary,
    team-based quality improvement leadership training program for clinicians: the partners clini-
    cal process improvement leadership program. Am J Med Qual. 2016. [epub ahead of print].
Rodrigue C, Seoane L, Gala RB, Piazza J, Amedee RG. Implementation of a faculty development
    curriculum emphasizing quality improvement and patient safety: results of a qualitative study.
    Ochsner J. 2013;13(3):319–21.
Sachdeva AK, Philibert I, Leach DC, Blair PG, Stewart LK, Rubinfeld IS, et al. Patient safety cur-
    riculum for surgical residency programs: results of a national consensus conference. Surgery.
    2007;141(4):427–41.
SCORE | General surgery resident curriculum portal [Internet]. The Surgical Council on Resident
    Education Inc.; c2009-16 [cited 2016 Jun 20. Available from: http://surgicalcore.org/.
Sellers MM, Hanson K, Schuller M, Sherman K, Kelz RR, Fryer J, et al. Development and partici-
    pant assessment of a practical quality improvement educational initiative for surgical residents.
    J Am Coll Surg. 2013a;216(6):1207–13, 1213.e1.
Sellers MM, Reinke CE, Kreider S, Meise C, Nelis K, Volpe A, et al. American College of Surgeons
    NSQIP: quality in-training initiative pilot study. J Am Coll Surg. 2013b;217(5):827–32.
Starr SR, Kautz JM, Sorita A, Thompson KM, Reed DA, Porter BL, et al. Quality improvement
    education for health professionals: a systematic review. Am J Med Qual. 2016;31(3):209–16.
Strayer RJ, Shy BD, Shearer PL. A novel program to improve patient safety by integrating peer
    review into the emergency medicine residency curriculum. J Emerg Med. 2014;47(6):696,701.e2.
Waits SA, Reames BN, Krell RW, Bryner B, Shih T, Obi AT, et al. Development of Team Action
    Projects in Surgery (TAPS): a multilevel team-based approach to teaching quality improve-
    ment. J Surg Educ. 2014;71(2):166–8.
Wong BM, Etchells EE, Kuper A, Levinson W, Shojania KG. Teaching quality improvement and
    patient safety to trainees: a systematic review. Acad Med. 2010;85(9):1425–39.

Chapter 10
Is 'Quality Science' Human Subjects Research?

Megan K. Applewhite and Peter Angelos

Abstract Physicians have an ethical obligation to their patients, institutions, and community to provide the highest quality of care possible. In the past 15 years, beginning with the Institute of Medicine's *To Err is Human* report (Kohn et al. To err is human: building a safer health system. Washington, DC: National Academies Press, 2000), Quality Improvement (QI) in surgery has been prioritized by national organizations, including the Centers for Medicare & Medicaid Services, the Center for Disease Control, the American College of Surgeons, and the Accreditation Council for Graduate Medical Education (ACGME). The aim of QI projects is to evaluate the quality of perioperative surgical care and design projects that modify systems and behavior within individual institutions to produce better patient outcomes.

Quality Improvement and Surgery

Physicians have an ethical obligation to their patients, institutions, and community to provide the highest quality of care possible. In the past 15 years, beginning with the Institute of Medicine's *To Err is Human* report (Kohn et al. 2000), Quality Improvement (QI) in surgery has been prioritized by national organizations, including the Centers for Medicare & Medicaid Services, the Center for Disease Control, the American College of Surgeons, and the Accreditation Council for Graduate Medical Education (ACGME). The aim of QI projects is to evaluate the quality of perioperative surgical care and design projects that modify systems and behavior within individual institutions to produce better patient outcomes.

M.K. Applewhite, MD
Department of Surgery and Alden March Bioethics Institute, Albany Medical College, Albany, NY, USA

P. Angelos, MD, PhD (✉)
Department of Surgery and MacLean Center for Clinical Medical Ethics, University of Chicago, Chicago, IL, USA
e-mail: pangelos@surgery.bsd.uchicago.edu

© Springer International Publishing Switzerland 2017
R.R. Kelz, S.L. Wong (eds.), *Surgical Quality Improvement*,
Success in Academic Surgery, DOI 10.1007/978-3-319-23356-7_10

This practice of employing QI projects into daily activities affects health care workers at every level, including surgeons and surgical trainees. Trainees are often the most immediately aware of inefficiencies and suboptimal systems practices in the local milieu, and, therefore, are in a unique position to affect change and make quality improvements in patient care. Residents are expected to initiate and execute QI projects during their training through the ACGME Clinical Learning Environment Review (CLER) a quality improvement focus area of the Next Accreditation System (Weiss et al. 2012). Due to the focus of these national organizations and the increasing importance of documenting and delivering efficient and high quality care, QI projects have become a regular practice in hospitals throughout the United States. The number of publications on this topic has risen dramatically over the past decade (Raval et al. 2014), and while this has increased the number of opportunities for academic involvement of physicians, residents, and students, it has also brought up the question of whether or not QI projects should be considered human subjects research.

As with any investigation, the safety and protection of the patient is of primary concern with QI projects, and it is imperative to employ the four core ethical principles of respect for autonomy, beneficence, nonmaleficence, and justice in these projects that govern the daily behavior of clinicians (Jonsen et al. 2015). Because of the wide breadth of these projects, the line has been blurred between "initiatives" and "research". There have been many attempts to distinguish differences and identify similarities of human subjects research (HSR) from QI projects in an effort to create guidelines in which to promote advancement of quality of care while still protecting patients. This chapter will address the ethical considerations in quality science (QS) and QI overall.

Definitions of Human Subjects Research and Quality Improvement Initiatives

In order to understand what research is, it is important to know where the current definition used by investigators today came from. The Nuremberg Code was established in 1947 after the "Doctors' Trial", in which 23 German physicians were investigated for war crimes and crimes against humanity in World War II concentration camps. Many of those accused were not punished for their crimes, as they argued that there was no clear law that outlined what type of experiments were legal and illegal. The Nuremberg Code was the first recognized international guideline written to address ethical aspects of human research, and it addressed topics including: informed consent, the absence of coercion, beneficence, and nonmaleficence. The Declaration of Helsinki built on this in 1964 and clarified that in research with human subjects: the risks should not exceed benefits, and protocols for investigations should be evaluated by outside review boards to ensure the safety of the participants. The Nuremburg Code and the Declaration of Helsinki are the basis for the Code of Federal Regulations Title 45 (Public Welfare) Part 46 (Protection of Human Subjects), of the United States Department of Health and Human Services regulations for human research (Services et al. 2009). The Federal Policy for the Protection of Human Subjects defines research in the "Common Rule" as "a systematic investigation, including research development, testing and evaluation, designed to develop or contribute to generalizable knowledge"(Services et al. 2009).

Protocols for HSR are subject to regulation by Institutional Review Boards (IRB) before studies are carried out, unless the IRB deems it to be exempt. HSR are systematic investigations that contribute to generalizable knowledge. Risks and benefits to the patients are variable and individual informed consent is necessary to thoroughly discuss these topics with the patient.

Quality improvement is "systematic, data-guided activities designed to bring about immediate improvements in health-care delivery in particular settings" (Baily et al. 2006). It is modifying intrinsic components of normal health care operations in the sense that it changes human performance to align with established best practices, but is not intended to answer a specific scientific inquiry or provide generalizable knowledge (Davidoff et al. 2009). The intention of QI projects are to optimize patient care with minimal risk to the patients, as they are in line with their interests and the interests of the community (Baily et al. 2006; Lynn et al. 2007). As such, QI project are not traditionally determined to be "research" and, therefore, neither require the approval of IRB, nor the need for individual informed consent. Funding for QI projects are typically internal to an institution, and they are implemented by changes in everyday clinical practice.

Quality Science and Research

There are several traits that are irrefutably different between HSR and QI projects, which is arguably why such QI projects have not, to date, required rigorous regulation or protocol-specific informed consent. However, because there is such a wide breadth of quality-related inquiries, there are times when the line between research and quality improvement becomes poorly defined and more regulation may become necessary.

Variation in QI projects and HSR protocol design illustrate differences in their fundamental makeup. For example, patients undergo rigorous evaluation to be determined if they should be included or excluded in a specific research investigation, and many are excluded if their profile does not precisely fit the mold that the investigators seek to study. This differs in QI projects, for which the goal to affect local change in a group of patients routinely encountered is more realistically tested and achieved if all patients of a specific disease process or part of the hospital are included in the study. Secondly, those patients included in research studies are often randomized, whereas those in QI projects are not (Raval et al. 2014). Additionally, the risks imposed on the participants of research studies are varied and there is no guaranteed benefit. In quality initiatives, the goal is a benefit to the patient and there is often minimal risk to them while trying to pursue that goal. The data being gathered for QI projects are not beyond routine patient care information that would have been gathered otherwise. The end goal of research studies is often to end in publication and generalizable knowledge, whereas QI projects are typically meant to be implemented locally.

When QI projects follow its classic definition, and patients have minimal risk and high likelihood of benefits, the overlap between HSR and QI work is small. However, this may be the minority of situations. Frequently, quality improvement initiatives vary dramatically from study to study such that some are potentially considered research endeavors. For example, there are many instances in which QI projects have a control group, thereby introducing a type of randomization. Although both the control and the investigational group may be within the standard of care, participants are still randomized. If this were a research study, the protocol would undergo IRB review and mandatory patient consent in order to allow for randomization. However, in QI work, this is not always a necessary requirement. Additionally, there are times when the investigator finds that a QI project may have external validity, and, in those cases, publication promotes the overall good of society and is pursued. While some institutions consider publication a requirement for IRB review and approval, others do not.

There have been many attempts to further clarify when QI becomes HSR (Raval et al. 2014; Baily et al. 2006; Lynn et al. 2007; Finkelstein et al. 2015); however, it may never be possible to establish firm universal guidelines that account for all possible investigations. As these investigations are intended to occur on the local level, ideally there should be institution-specific guidelines and regulation to discern if any given QI project falls on the spectrum of research.

Regulation and Oversight

Oversight of research includes approval from the IRB and patient informed consent. With HIPPA, if the institution is covered by Privacy Rule, QI activities do not require patient authorization. In many institutions, QI efforts are included under the blanket consent that the patient signs when consenting to care in the hospital. In these cases, and when the QI project poses minimal risk in an effort to improve local care standards, involving the IRB may not be cost effective and could slow down progress of the project.

Even for the most basic QI projects, it is prudent to have a hospital oversight committee that is responsible for determining when a QI project qualifies as research and, in the case that it does, formal oversight and informed consent should be carried out. In order to most efficiently and effectively review QI research, IRBs need to be staffed with a reviewer specifically focused on quality initiatives, and the application and implementation of QI project protocols can benefit from a certain amount of flexibility for dynamic intervention, which can facilitate the success of a quality initiative. Hospital oversight committees designed by each institution to oversee QI projects safely and appropriately can guide study design and implementation to minimize risk to patients and simultaneously aid in the identification of when these projects become research.

Ethical Responsibilities in Quality Science Initiatives

The intention of QI is to take suboptimal hospital or clinic practices and improve them such that the standard of quality is optimized. Theoretically, as previously mentioned, this imposes minimal risk on the patient and ultimately results in significant benefit. As long as this is true, and QI projects are a benefit to society, it is the ethical responsibility of the physician and other healthcare workers to engage in quality related initiatives. Similarly, as one who will ultimately benefit, patients should readily participate in QI projects that do not carry risk. This is distinctively different in intention than a human subjects-related research endeavor, in which a project is intended to provide "generalizable knowledge", or, to investigate subjects to generate previously unknown qualitative or quantitative scientific results.

QI projects are primarily designed with clear benefit intended in terms of safety, quality, efficiency, satisfaction, or cost (Raval et al. 2014). While engaging in QI projects is the responsibility of physicians and other healthcare workers, it does not mean that these initiatives should be undertaken without patient safety considerations, cost considerations, or hospital oversight/regulation. There are several ethical considerations in quality improvement projects as outlined by the Hastings Center Report in 2006 (Baily et al. 2006). At times, QI projects can have unintended consequences and cause harm to patients if the intervention is not appropriately implemented or not utilized for the proper patient population. Additionally, QI projects may waste resources that are scarce and end up being costly without any ultimate benefits to the patients.

Insofar as physicians have an obligation to community, they have a commitment to improve healthcare to the highest standard, but engaging in these initiatives can be confusing because it is not clear when it is determined to be research or when the IRB should be involved. Some argue that actively pursuing improvement in the quality of practice and outcomes is a necessary component of professionalism (Millenson 2003) and to not engage actively in pursuit of the quality standard directly negatively impacts patients (McGlynn et al. 2003). However, the lack of clarity for the necessity of oversight can make this a challenge. An additional challenge is raised in the case that the initiative is successful and the physician believes it to have external validity and wishes to publish results.

Patients also have an ethical obligation to participate in QI projects. They have benefitted from previous quality improvement efforts and to better the greater good and future patient care, they have an obligation to participate if they will encounter minimal risk and potentially significant benefit. Patients should have a thorough understanding of the project and should be updated routinely on the progress of the work.

Conclusion

The answer to the question 'Is Quality Science research?' is: sometimes. The goal of research is to discover and disseminate knowledge, whereas, the goal of quality improvement project is to change performance (Davidoff and Batalden 2005).

Fundamental to the determination of whether or not quality science is HSR is understanding key components of what makes a project 'research.' If initiatives pose minimal risks to the subjects, are conducted to bring routine healthcare operations to the standard of care, and are focused on enhancing patient care at the local level, they are considered QI projects and may be carried out under hospital-designed oversight committee and after thorough explanation to the patient. However, the protocol is oftentimes not clear, and should be reviewed by an oversight committee to determine whether or not it should undergo formal IRB review. Hospital oversight committees are valuable to evaluate QI project protocols, determine risk to the patient, relationship of the project to standard of care, and what population the initiative is intended to impact. Ultimately, QI work and HSR are not mutually exclusive, and it is the responsibility of the investigator to critically appraise the protocol and involve oversight committees as appropriate in the best interests of the patients affected.

What is fundamental and should be universally employed is high quality patient education. Teaching patients about what QI is and informing them about ongoing hospital QI projects is imperative for disclosure and for respecting the patient's right to know. At the time of the administration of the generalized hospital consent, patients should be informed explicitly about the regular performance of QIP in each hospital; and, their likely involvement in the process.

References

Baily MA, et al. The ethics of using QI methods to improve health care quality and safety. Hastings Cent Rep. 2006;36(4):S1–40.

Davidoff F, Batalden P. Toward stronger evidence on quality improvement. Draft publication guidelines: the beginning of a consensus project. Qual Saf Health Care. 2005;14(5):319–25.

Davidoff F, et al. Publication guidelines for quality improvement studies in health care: evolution of the SQUIRE project. BMJ. 2009;338:a3152.

Finkelstein JA, et al. Oversight on the borderline: quality improvement and pragmatic research. Clin Trials. 2015;12(5):457–66.

Jonsen AR, Siegler M, Winslade WJ. Clinical ethics: a practical approach to ethical decisions in clinical medicine. 8th ed. New York: McGraw-Hill Education; 2015.

Kohn LT, Corrigan JM, Donaldson MS, editors. To err is human: building a safer health system. Washington, DC: National Academies Press; 2000.

Lynn J, et al. The ethics of using quality improvement methods in health care. Ann Intern Med. 2007;146(9):666–73.

McGlynn EA, et al. The quality of health care delivered to adults in the United States. N Engl J Med. 2003;348(26):2635–45.

Millenson ML. The silence. Health Aff (Millwood). 2003;22(2):103–12.

Raval MV, et al. Distinguishing QI projects from human subjects research: ethical and practical considerations. Bull Am Coll Surg. 2014;99(7):21–7.

Services U.S.D.o.H.H. Code of federal regulations. Title 45: public welfare, part 46: protection of human subjects 2009 January 15, 2010. Cited 15 Feb 2016. Available from: http://www.hhs.gov/ohrp/humansubjects/guidance/45cfr46.html.

Weiss KB, Wagner R, Nasca TJ. Development, testing, and implementation of the ACGME Clinical Learning Environment Review (CLER) program. J Grad Med Educ. 2012;4(3):396–8.

Chapter 11
Academic Careers in Quality Improvement

Brad S Oriel and Kamal M.F. Itani

Abstract Codman introduced the modern concept of quality improvement (QI) in surgery in the late nineteenth century. The assessment of surgical outcomes helped pave the way for provider and hospital comparisons on complications and mortality after various procedures. Later, mortality and morbidity were risk adjusted based on patient factors, which allowed for comparisons across different populations and environments. The science behind risk adjustment was the pillar of academic career development for surgeons in the twentieth century. The field later incorporated patient safety, patient satisfaction, quality of life after surgery, long-term functional outcome, access to care, disparities and cost. As such, the field evolved from risk adjusted mortality and morbidity to the broader field of surgical outcomes. Adding infrastructure, processes, coordination of care, staff education and culture transformed the field into the broader arena of health services. Surgeons interested in any of these areas can endeavor into scholarly activities and have a lasting impact. Over the last two decades, the health services research and practice derived from nurturing young surgeons and supporting them through their career development has resulted in improved systems, provider performance and patient care. The founders of surgical QI would be proud of the field's rapid and far-reaching expansion and the enthusiasm of academic surgeons of all ages to pursue new related ventures. With the availability of health services research fellowships and the multitude of institutional, regional, national and international programs serving the surgical patient, careers dedicated to quality improvement present many opportunities for growth and future leadership in surgical care.

Introduction

Passion and scholarly activities are the tenets of an academic career in any field of interest. In medicine, areas for academic growth broadly include the basic, clinical and translational sciences, education and health services research. This chapter

B.S. Oriel, MD
VA Boston Healthcare System, Tufts University School of Medicine, Boston, MA, USA

K.M.F. Itani, MD, FACS (✉)
VA Boston Healthcare System, Boston University and Harvard Medical School, Boston, MA, USA
e-mail: kamal.itani@va.gov

© Springer International Publishing Switzerland 2017
R.R. Kelz, S.L. Wong (eds.), *Surgical Quality Improvement*,
Success in Academic Surgery, DOI 10.1007/978-3-319-23356-7_11

$$Value = \frac{Quality\ (Access + Outcome + Functional\ Status + Satisfaction + Quality\ of\ Life)}{Cost}$$

Fig. 11.1 Value of care

focuses on health services research and the path that one can follow to develop an academic career in surgical quality improvement.

One way health services evaluates quality is through outcome measures. Standardized definitions of variables and metrics used in calculating outcome measures ensure their validity. Traditional outcome measures include mortality and select morbidities within 30 days of surgery. Mortality and morbidity data have been used to establish trends over time, which in turn have helped to drive improvement, and compare practices and facilities. Other quality metrics continue to gain popularity and include patient access to care, satisfaction, long-term functional outcome, safety, disparities, cost of care and health-related quality of life (HRQOL). The International Society for Quality of Life Research defines the latter as a subjective measure comprised of one's physical and occupational function, psychological state, social interactions and somatic sensations. With the increase in health care costs, value, or the ratio of quality over cost, is yet another metric, which has gained momentum (Fig. 11.1).

The scholarly activities associated with these areas of focus begin with identifying experts in the field who can mentor and collaborate in the area identified as an interest. Databases and observational studies are used to gather preliminary data that are subsequently used to develop research proposals and to obtain funding. Obtaining funding is the most difficult yet most crucial step in the early stages of career development. Funding engenders more funding, results in personal growth, leads to additional experiences and drives scholarly work. This will then lead to expertise and the ability to mentor younger surgeons with an interest in the same field.

Mentorship

The identification and declaration of a strong interest in health services sets the foundation for a career in that field. Selecting a focus within that field often occurs during one's clinical training and may stem from a personal or patient experience, from reading on an engaging topic, or from speaking with a colleague or supervisor. The field is very broad and narrowing the spectrum in which one nurtures an idea is crucial. Finding a mentor is the next most important step after focusing on an area of interest. This person is typically a well-funded and well-respected investigator capable of collaboration and tutelage. Interacting with local faculty, reading publications within a chosen focus and contacting investigators will help in identifying a mentor. In addition, it will help to construct a network of collaborators in fields other than medicine such as psychology, sociology, economics, and system engineering, all of which are integral within the multidisciplinary field of health services.

Advanced Studies in Health Services Research

As a means to conduct more methodological research, new investigators often pursue an advanced or supplementary degree. The Master of Public Health degree, for instance, allows for in-depth focus in specific areas: clinical effectiveness, epidemiology, biostatistics, global health, health management and health policy. Other advanced degrees include a Doctor of Philosophy in biological sciences, public health, biostatistics, health policy, health services, or population health sciences. Additional opportunities available to tailor one's research skills include the National Cancer Institute funded postdoctoral training program in implementation science and the American College of Surgeons (ACS)-sponsored Clinical Scholars in Residence program. In this program, the Scholar participates in ongoing quality improvement initiatives and guideline development with ACS programs, while having the opportunity to obtain a Master of Science degree in clinical investigation, health services and outcomes research, or healthcare quality and safety. The program specifically targets candidates wishing to focus on national surgical healthcare issues. The ACS also hosts the Clinical Trials Methods Course and Outcomes Research Course, which offer didactics and skills-based labs. Other surgical specialty organizations have duplicated these courses and made them available to interested specialty surgeons.

Further opportunities for fellowship, course work and ancillary training are present within the Department of Veterans Affairs (VA). The VA Interprofessional Fellowship Program in Patient Safety is a 1-year fellowship within the Office of Academic Affiliations and the National Center for Patient Safety designed for post-residency trained physicians and postdoctoral or post-master degree trained health professionals; it provides education in patient safety practice and leadership. The VA also offers the Quality Scholars Fellowship Program, a 2-year post-residency fellowship for physicians and pre- or post-doctoral fellowship for nurses. It focuses on improving health care delivery, health systems organization and management, and health professions education. Other learning opportunities exist through the Professional Health Informatics Training and VA Health Informatics Certificate Program.

The Surgical Outcomes Club (SOC), together with the Association for Academic Surgery (AAS) and Society of University Surgeons, offer a variety of monthly didactic sessions. Similarly, HarvardX and the Institute for Health Care Improvement offer an online course on Translating Innovations or Evidence into Practice. The SOC also sponsors, through the SOC Research Fellowship Program, the Michael Zinner Health Services Research Fellowship, a 1-year fellowship, which pairs a young investigator with an SOC member mentor. Lastly, the AAS offers two courses: Fundamentals of Surgical Research and Early Career Development. Ultimately, supplementing ones knowledge with information built from the public health perspective will aid in drafting hypotheses, study design, study execution, biostatistical analysis, and implementation into clinical practice. An advanced degree provides necessary knowledge, builds confidence and allows practice in disseminating information at all levels to influence care.

Funding

With a foundation set, initial investigative work will take advantage of available databases to perform studies pertaining to the area of interest. This work aids in the preparation of future prospective studies and provides preliminary evidence needed to support funding applications. Initial funding opportunities are often modest and may take the form of research training awards, career development awards, career transition awards or global leader awards. With persistence and careful planning, a novice investigator may quickly find their research supported by one large or multiple smaller awards. All together, these awards catalyze career development and allow for the pursuit of more substantial funding.

Obtaining the resources necessary to engage in research is important and challenging. Grant funding is available from multiple sources. The Veterans Integrated Service Network funds a Career Development Award (CDA) for 2-years of salary support to a mentored junior investigator who expresses a clear commitment to a VA career. Similarly, the VA Health Services Research and Development Service (HSR&D) promotes Veteran-centric projects and hosts a Research Career Development Program designed to provide mentoring for junior researchers. A mentored CDA provides salary support to early-career investigators with the goal of developing them into independent VA-funded health services researchers. Within the VA, HSR&D funds 19 Centers of Innovation (COINs), each of which includes one or more focused areas of health services research. The VA HSR&D also awards funding through an Investigator Initiated Research program, which contributes to the quality, effectiveness and efficiency of VA health care. Furthermore, the Quality Enhancement Research Initiative aims to translate research evidence into clinical practice.

The Patient-Centered Outcomes Research Institute (PCORI), an independent nonprofit nongovernmental organization, is another resource. PCORI is funded by the PCOR Trust Fund established by Congress in 2010 and is fed by the general fund of the Treasury, transfers from the Centers for Medicare and Medicaid trust funds and the PCOR fee assessed on private and self-insured health plans. Available research funding is geared towards helping investigators conduct comparative clinical effectiveness research (CER), with a focus on patient-centered care. In addition, PCORI will also support research focused on improving the methods used to conduct CER.

The Agency for Healthcare Research and Quality (AHRQ) sponsors multiple CDAs in support of investigators in the field of health services research. The following K awards provide salary and research support for early career clinicians and research scientists for a period of 3–5 years: Mentored Clinical Scientist Development Awards (K08), PCOR Mentored Clinical Investigator Award (K08) and PCOR Mentored Research Scientist Development Award (K01).

The National Institutes of Health research training and career development program hosts many awards accessible to postdoctoral researchers and clinical residents, as well to independent researchers who are actively or have recently transferred to positions as investigators, faculty members, clinician scientists or scientific team leaders in industry.

Other awards exist through professional societies in the form of seed or supplemental funding to aid in a project's initial development and progress sufficient to attain larger awards. As an example, the ACS offers the Franklin H. Martin, MD, FACS Faculty Research Fellowship honoring the ACS founder and the Thomas R. Russell, MD, FACS Faculty Research Fellowship designated to support research into improving surgical outcomes. These are 2-year awards, which offer $40,000 per year to assist a surgeon in the establishment of a new and independent research program. For those investigators who are mid-career, the ACS also offers the Jacobson Promising Investigator Award, which recognizes surgeons conducting research who are contributing to and advancing surgical practice and patient safety. The Association for Academic Surgery Foundation, the American Surgical Association Foundation, the Surgical Infection Society Foundation, as well as other specialty organizations, offer similar awards.

One additional resource, though not specific to surgery, is the Josiah Macy Jr Foundation. The Foundation, first established in 1930, fosters innovation in health professional education in order to help align their education with contemporary health needs and a changing health care system. It supports projects committed to providing new curriculum content for health professional education, including patient safety, QI, systems performance and professionalism.

Databases, Clinical Research and Available Resources

In the initial stages of investigation, young investigators formulate ideas, identify questions and attempt to answer those questions with the use of databases and registries. These resources allow for prospective and real time entry of data and prospective follow up or retrospective review of patients' postoperative courses. In prospectively collected data, the variables are carefully defined a priori, and as such, result in a very complete database with standardized variables and few missing fields. Analyses may focus on local data or perhaps be inclusive of larger healthcare systems such as the Veterans Affairs Surgical Quality Improvement Program (VASQIP), or its counterpart in the private sector, the American College of Surgeons National Surgical Quality Improvement Project (ACS-NSQIP). Together with data from the Medicare Coverage Database (Centers for Medicare and Medicaid Services; CMS), the National Cancer Institute's Surveillance, Epidemiology, and End Results Program (SEER data) and the ACS trauma and cancer databases, these large repositories allow for data selection, manipulation, analysis and comparison. Landmark publications from these databases are frequently cited (see suggested reading section) and their importance cannot be overstated. Training mentored junior faculty on "big data" manipulation and analysis is a key component to their development as independent investigators.

Findings originating from retrospective analyses may be used in the pursuit of diverse funding opportunities required to plan prospective observational studies and randomized clinical trials. Alternatively, databases can be used to conduct point-of-care pragmatic studies through randomization and long-term follow up. Analysis of databases can also help in the development of evidence difficult to obtain through other means yet necessary for guidelines and consensus statements.

Leadership and Initiatives

As a leader, one may affect local, regional, national or international practices and policies. At the local level, the impact of an academic leader may extend from serving as a mentor to postdoctoral fellows engaging in health services, outcome and QI research, to serving as a champion in health care improvement projects within a hospital.

Deciding to focus on resolving quality issues or poor outcomes such as surgical site infection, or high rates of major cardiac events after surgery might be the first step in leading a quality improvement project. This often requires a review of best practices and the development of care bundles or clinical guidelines. Implementation of any intervention is best accompanied by data collection before and after the intervention to evaluate the impact of that intervention. This by itself can lead to several presentations and publications. Pre-implementation data collection can also entail the review of large databases with opportunities to study risk factors and their contribution to the outcome. Departmental leaders and quality managers are always looking for volunteers to address those issues; it represents a tremendous opportunity for young faculty to engage in such projects at the local level to grow and to engage in scholarly activities. This in turn will afford credibility when requesting funding or applying for grants to answer specific questions in quality improvement. Other opportunities may then follow at the departmental or hospital level. It is not uncommon for interested individuals to become the lead hospital champion for the NSQIP program, a departmental quality manager or vice chair for quality within the department or even move to bigger responsibilities within the hospital to tackle issues that go beyond surgical care and may affect the whole health care system. These contributions are recognized locally and noticed regionally and internationally, especially when accompanied by scholarly work and will allow for promotion from assistant to associate to full professor.

At the regional level, many states have initiated a surgical quality collaborative with the goal of performing statewide healthcare research to improve quality and reduce disparities. Program success was illustrated first in Michigan in 2005 and later by Tennessee in 2008. Another program first piloted in 2005 and later expanded in 2008, the Surgical Care and Outcomes Assessment Program (SCOAP), is a Washington-state approved Coordinated Quality Improvement Program. It is operated under the Foundation for Health Care Quality but its research and development work is performed by the University of Washington's Department of Surgery's

Surgical Outcomes Research Center. It is a statewide performance surveillance program targeting safety, quality, efficiency and appropriateness of surgical care, which is physician-led (including leadership of the state chapter of the ACS) and voluntary. Over 12 additional regional collaborative groups fall under the ACS-NSQIP umbrella (Table 11.1). Within each collaborative lie opportunities for leadership gained through election.

Institutional level efforts often serve as a foundation for change at the regional and national levels. Similar to pieces of a national healthcare system puzzle, if each of the academic centers works to improve surgical safety and outcomes locally, regional- and nation-wide impact is possible through collaboration among these centers and information dissemination. For example, AHRQ collaborates with the U.S. Department of Health and Human Services (USDHHS) to produce evidence to improve healthcare safety, quality and accessibility, and to make it equitable and affordable. A 21-member National Advisory Council for Healthcare Research and Quality offers advice on AHRQ's research trajectory to the Secretary of the USDHHS. All members are private-sector experts and represent healthcare plans, providers, purchasers, consumers and researchers.

The National Quality Forum (NQF) serves an important role in the sponsorship and endorsement of quality measures in the United States; the federal government and private sector payers utilize information directed by the Measure Applications Partnership in quality, payment and accountability programs. A Board of Directors and five Board Committees oversee the NQF. The CDC's National Healthcare Safety Network serves over 14,500 medical facilities by tracking healthcare-associated infections and is the system used to satisfy CMS' infection reporting requirements.

Not-for-profit institutions like the Joint Commission (JC) serve to improve public health by evaluating institutions and ensuring safe, high quality, and effective care is being practiced. Finally, collaborations such as the University HealthSystem Consortium (UHC) foster hospital comparisons by coordinating the sharing of clinical, safety, operational and financial data of over 200 hospitals. These data are used

Table 11.1 Regional ACS-NSQIP collaboratives

Canadian National surgical quality improvement collaborative
Connecticut surgical quality coalition
Florida surgical care initiative
Georgia surgical quality collaborative
Illinois surgical quality improvement collaborative
Northern California surgical quality collaborative
Nebraska collaborative
Ontario collaborative
Oregon NSQIP consortium
Pennsylvania NSQIP consortium
Tennessee surgical quality collaborative
Upstate New York surgical quality initiative
Virginia surgical quality collaborative

to improve quality, safety and cost-effectiveness. The UHC offers councils composed of representatives from UHC member organizations and the ACS overheads many regional collaborative organizations as well as the Surgical Quality Alliance.

Giants in Quality Improvement

More experience, funding and publication yields leadership opportunities, but these are fraught with countless barriers and resistance. Research in QI challenges by its very nature the fabric of the current system in which we all work. Disruption of a systems' framework, or scrutinizing department, specialty-level or individual outcomes is often met with apprehension or opposition. One such example lies in the story of Dr. Ernest Amory Codman, renowned founder of outcomes measurement with a lifelong pursuit of an "end results system of hospitalization standardization."

Between the late nineteenth and early twentieth centuries, Dr. Codman studied at Harvard Medical School and later became a member of the Harvard faculty while practicing surgery at Massachusetts General Hospital (MGH). He subsequently established his own 12-bed hospital after resigning from MGH in 1914 because the hospital refused to accept his idea to promote surgeons based on competence rather than seniority. His resignation was also requested from the Suffolk District Medical Society's Surgical Section following their meeting in 1915 during which he displayed a controversial cartoon of an ostrich with its head in the sand satirizing his view of the MGH approach to quality and safety. Despite these setbacks, he is recognized for instituting morbidity and mortality conferences as well as for serving a critical role in the founding of the ACS along with its Committee on Hospital Standardization, now the familiar JC. From his pioneering efforts, QI has grown into a multi-national, publicly transparent and all-encompassing field. The End Result System, though not popular during his lifetime, is founded in the DNA of current QI systems and Dr. Codman is credited with setting the modern stage for patient-centered quality based surgery.

In 1996, the JC established the Ernest Amory Codman Award to recognize Dr. Codman's courage, efforts, and contributions to quality improvement. Two of the awardees illustrate many of the principles presented above.

The first one, Dr. Avedis Donabedian was born in Beirut, Lebanon in 1919. His medical career took him to Ramallah, Jerusalem and England in addition to doing his studies at the American University of Beirut. While in Beirut, he was given the opportunity to obtain a Master of Public Health degree from Harvard in 1955 through a scholarship from the school's Dean. His work ultimately led him to the University of Michigan School of Public Health where he devised his well-known conceptual quality framework of structure, process, and outcomes (Fig. 11.2). These components, respectively defined as the healthcare services environment, the tasks involved in the provision of medical services, and measured outcomes of the study at hand, drove changes in social attitudes and healthcare-related public policies. His work culminated in the receipt of the Ernest A. Codman award in 1997. He also received

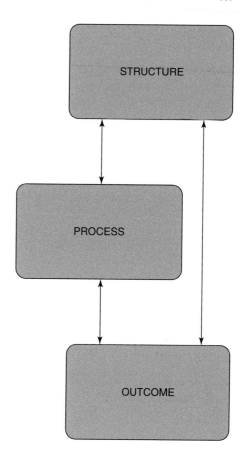

Fig. 11.2 Donabedian conceptual quality framework

the Sedgwick Award in 1999 given by the American Public Health Association who also established an Annual Avedis Donabedian Health Care Quality Award.

The second one, Dr. Shukri Khuri, was born in 1943 in Jerusalem. He received his medical degree from the American University of Beirut and further trained at Johns Hopkins and the Mayo Clinic. In 1976, he was recruited to Harvard and the Boston VA hospital where he researched cardiac perfusion and tissue preservation. He established the Boston VA hospital as a "Center of Excellence" in Cardiac Surgery, and also served for 20 years as Chief of the Surgical Service. Together with Jennifer Daley, M.D. and William Henderson, Ph.D., he was instrumental in the development of NSQIP within the Department of Veterans Affairs and its validity within the private sector. In 1998, Dr. Khuri was awarded the Frank Brown Berry Prize in Federal Medicine for his work in cardiac surgery and surgical care quality. For his NSQIP work extending 16 years, together with over 20 years of work in surgical QI, the JC presented the Ernest A. Codman Award to Dr. Khuri posthumously in 2008. This honor recognized his achievements in the use of process and outcome measures to improve organization performance and, ultimately, the quality and safety of care provided to the public.

Conclusion

A career in academic surgical QI has the potential to be a rewarding experience. It requires a self-motivated leader, an inquisitive thinker, an empathetic personality, and a strong collaborator, mentor and public advocate. Given the evolving complexities of health care systems and continued advances in medical care and medical technology, more experts in health services and quality improvement will be needed. In addition, with financial penalties imposed on healthcare systems for comparatively poorer outcomes and evolving pay-for-performance initiatives, QI research and expertise will become increasingly necessary, opening up more opportunities for academic surgical careers in this area.

Suggested Readings

Daley J, Khuri SF, Henderson W, et al. Risk adjustment of the postoperative morbidity rate for the comparative assessment of the quality of surgical care: results of the National Veterans Affairs Surgical Risk study. J Am Coll Surg. 1997;185(4):328–40.

Donabedian A. The quality of care. How can it be assessed? JAMA. 1988;260(12):1743–8.

Khuri SF, Henderson WG, Daley J, et al. Successful implementation of the Department of Veterans Affairs' National Surgical Quality Improvement Program in the private sector: the Patient Safety in Surgery study. Ann Surg. 2008;248(2):329–36.

Rodkey GV, Itani KM. Evaluation of healthcare quality: a tale of three giants. Am J Surg. 2009;198(5 Suppl):S3–8.

Chapter 12
National Quality Improvement: Federal Regulation, Public Reporting, and the Surgeon

Jason B. Liu, Bruce L. Hall, and Clifford Y. Ko

Abstract A paradigm shift in the structure and delivery of healthcare in the United States occurred on March 23, 2010 when President Barack Obama signed the Patient Protection and Affordable Care Act (PPACA or ACA), which was subsequently upheld against challenges in the United States Supreme Court in June 2012. Now in the post-ACA era as the various provisions of the law move through stages of implementation, it is critical for surgeons to understand the moving pieces. A central tenet of the ACA is to foster quality in healthcare by holding healthcare providers, both at the institutional and physician levels, accountable for the care they provide to patients. To this end, the Secretary of the Department and Health and Human Services (HHS) developed the United States National Quality Strategy (NQS) with a core aim to "measure care delivery and outcomes using consistent, nationally-endorsed measures to provide information that is timely, actionable, and meaningful to both providers and patients." Fostering surgical quality, as discussed in this book, has been a doctrine of the surgical profession long before the enactment of the ACA. Nevertheless, these regulatory changes and additions are likely here to stay, and surgeons must understand the impact of these national healthcare quality initiatives.

J.B. Liu, MD (✉)
Department of Research and Optimal Patient Care,
American College of Surgeons, Chicago, IL, USA
e-mail: jliu@facs.org

B.L. Hall, MD, PhD, MBA, FACS
Department of Research and Optimal Patient Care,
American College of Surgeons, Chicago, IL, USA

Department of Surgery, Washington University in St. Louis,
St. Louis, MO, USA

C.Y. Ko, MD, MS, MSHS, FACS
Department of Research and Optimal Patient Care,
American College of Surgeons, Chicago, IL, USA

Department of Surgery, University of California Los Angeles,
David Geffen School of Medicine,
Veterans Affairs Greater Los Angeles Healthcare System,
Los Angeles, CA, USA

© Springer International Publishing Switzerland 2017   111
R.R. Kelz, S.L. Wong (eds.), *Surgical Quality Improvement*,
Success in Academic Surgery, DOI 10.1007/978-3-319-23356-7_12

Introduction

A paradigm shift in the structure and delivery of healthcare in the United States occurred on March 23, 2010 when President Barack Obama signed the Patient Protection and Affordable Care Act (PPACA or ACA), which was subsequently upheld against challenges in the United States Supreme Court in June 2012. Now in the post-ACA era as the various provisions of the law move through stages of implementation, it is critical for surgeons to understand the moving pieces. A central tenet of the ACA is to foster quality in healthcare by holding healthcare providers, both at the institutional and physician levels, accountable for the care they provide to patients. To this end, the Secretary of the Department and Health and Human Services (HHS) developed the United States National Quality Strategy (NQS) with a core aim to "measure care delivery and outcomes using consistent, nationally-endorsed measures to provide information that is timely, actionable, and meaningful to both providers and patients" (U.S. Department of Health and Human Services 2011). Fostering surgical quality, as discussed in this book, has been a doctrine of the surgical profession long before the enactment of the ACA. Nevertheless, these regulatory changes and additions are likely here to stay, and surgeons must understand the impact of these national healthcare quality initiatives.

This chapter discusses in brief surgical quality improvement initiatives at the national level with specific emphasis on the surgeon rather than the hospital. Current regulatory efforts from federal agencies, designed to influence the delivery of high quality surgical care, are discussed in conjunction with national surgeon-specific public reporting efforts that might improve the delivery of high quality surgical care.

National Programs

Current Programs

Centers for Medicare and Medicaid Services

Currently, the Centers for Medicare and Medicaid Services (CMS) operates on three provisions set forth by the ACA to create incentives for quality: the Physician Quality Reporting System (PQRS), the Electronic Health Records (EHR) Incentive Program (also known as "Meaningful Use"), and the Value-Based Modifier Program (VBM). Although full discussion of how each individual component affects reimbursement is beyond the scope of this chapter, we will discuss briefly how these affect surgeons as quality initiatives (Fig. 12.1) (Centers for Medicare and Medicaid Services2016; American College of Surgeons 2016). These individual programs will be replaced by or incorporated into the nascent Merit-based Incentive Payment System (MIPS) effort by 2017–2019, as further described below.

The PQRS began in 2007 and was the first national program designed by CMS to link the reporting of quality data to individual physician payment. Focus on PQRS intensified when the ACA replaced the incentives for physicians participating in the program with penalties for providers who do not submit qualifying PQRS data.

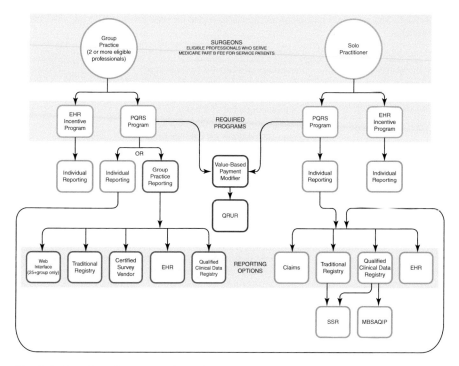

Fig. 12.1 Overview of current Medicare Quality Programs prior to MIPS implementation

Incentives were shifted to the VBM program. There were 284 quality measures for which providers may choose to submit data in 2016 (Centers for Medicare and Medicaid Services 2016). These measures are categorized using the six quality domains set forth by the NQS. CMS allows surgeons to submit PQRS data through several methods, including claims-based reporting, qualified clinical data registry (QCDR), direct submission from an EHR or other IT system vendor, and the Group Practice Reporting Option (GPRO) web interface. Each of these reporting options has criteria for satisfactorily reporting on the quality measures. Table 12.1 describes the 2015 PQRS General Surgery Measures Group. The American College of Surgeons (ACS) developed the Surgeon Specific Registry (SSR) to allow tracking and assessment of individual surgeon performance, both for surgeon self-improvement and for fulfillment of new regulatory requirements. The ACS SSR has been approved by CMS as one of the several QCDRs that can be used for measure submission.

The VBM provides for differential payment to a physician or group of physicians under the Medicare Physician Fee Schedule (PFS) and is based on the quality of care furnished relative to the cost during a performance period. Quality is determined as a composite score using the measures defined for PQRS. CMS uses five total per capita cost measures and the Medicare Spending per Beneficiary (MSPB) measure to determine a cost composite. The value-based modified amount is then calculated using the interplay between the quality composite score and the cost composite score.

The Health Information Technology for Economic and Clinical Health (HITECH) Act was enacted under the American Recovery and Reinvestment Act (ARRA) on

Table 12.1 Measures may change on an annual basis, and the ones for year 2015 are provided as an example

Measure title	PQRS #	Description	NQS domain	Type
Documentation of Current Medications in the Medical Record	130	Percentage of visits for patients aged 18 years and older for which the eligible professional attests to documenting a list of current medications using all immediate resources available on the date of the encounter. This list must include ALL known prescriptions, over-the-counters, herbals, and vitamin/mineral/dietary (nutritional) supplements AND must contain the medications' name, dosage, frequency and route of administration	Patient Safety	Process
Preventive Care and Screening: Tobacco Use: Screening and Cessation Intervention	226	Percentage of patients aged 18 years and older who were screened for tobacco use one or more times within 24 months AND who received cessation counseling intervention if identified as a tobacco user	Community/Population Health	Process
Anastomotic Leak Intervention	354	Percentage of patients aged 18 years and older who required an anastomotic leak intervention following gastric bypass or colectomy surgery	Patient Safety	Outcome
Unplanned Reoperation within the 30 day Postoperative Period	355	Percentage of patients aged 18 years and older who had any unplanned reoperation within the 30 day postoperative period	Patient Safety	Outcome
Unplanned Hospital Readmission within 30 days of Principal Procedure	356	Percentage of patients aged 18 years and older who had an unplanned hospital readmission within 30 days of principal procedure	Effective Clinical Care	Outcome
Surgical Site Infection (SSI)	357	Percentage of patients aged 18 years and older who had a surgical site infection (SSI)	Effective Clinical Care	Outcome
Patient-Centered Surgical Risk Assessment and Communication	358	Percentage of patients who underwent a non-emergency surgery who had their personalized risks of postoperative complications assessed by their surgical team prior to surgery using a clinical data-based, patient-specific risk calculator and who received personal discussion of those risks with the surgeon	Person and Caregiver-Centered Experience and Outcomes	Process

February 17, 2009, and was created to stimulate the adoption of health information technology by providing financial incentives to eligible health professions who demonstrate "meaningful use" of electronic health records. To receive an EHR incentive payment, providers have to show that they are "meaningfully using" their certified EHR technology by meeting certain measurement thresholds that range from recording patient information as structured data to exchanging summary care records.

It is important to note that for many CMS programs, the performance period typically predates the payment period by about 2 years. In other words, measured performance in the calendar year 2015 can affect reimbursements, incentives, and penalties levied in 2017. This also means that if there are performance problems in certain areas, it will take a minimum of 2 years to correct the performance and have that reflected in reimbursements. Providers cannot afford to further delay identification and correction of problems.

Agency for Healthcare Research and Quality

The Agency for Healthcare Research and Quality (AHRQ) is one of the 11 operating divisions of HHS alongside CMS. Established in 1989, the AHRQ supports research designed to improve the quality of healthcare, reduce its costs, address patient safety and medical errors, and broaden access to medical services. A number of centers within AHRQ specialize in major areas of healthcare research such as quality improvement and patient safety, outcomes and effectiveness of care, clinical practice and technology assessment, as well as healthcare organization and delivery systems. AHRQ is also a major source of funding and technical assistance for health services researchers and research training. It publishes the Annual National Healthcare Quality and Disparities report, which follows trends in the effectiveness of care, patient safety, and other factors.

The AHRQ also maintains the Consumer Assessment of Healthcare Providers and Systems (CAHPS) survey, which provides valid assessments of patients' experience of care in hospitals on topics such as communication with health care professionals and coordination of care. Currently, results of the CAHPS surveys are integrated into the PQRS and VBM programs, and results are publically reported on both the *Hospital Compare* and *Physician Compare* websites.

The Consumer Assessment of Healthcare Providers and Systems Surgical Care Survey (S-CAHPS) was sponsored by the ACS and developed in partnership with other surgical organizations. It expands the current CAHPS survey by incorporating three phases of surgical care including informed consent, anesthesia care, and postoperative follow up, and addresses both the ambulatory and inpatient surgical settings. However, S-CAHPS has not yet been implemented widely across the nation. Other programs maintained by the AHRQ include the Medical Expenditure Panel Survey (MEPS) and the Healthcare Cost and Utilization Project (HCUP). The National (Nationwide) Inpatient Sample (NIS), for example, is a publically available inpatient health care data base developed for the HCUP that has been used extensively for observational studies in the surgical literature (Healthcare Cost and Utilization Project 2015).

Patient-Centered Outcomes Research Institute

To implement the NQS priority of "ensuring that each person and family members are engaged as partners in their care," the ACA established the Patient-Centered Outcomes Research Institute (PCORI) as an independent, non-profit organization. Authorized by Congress in 2010, its mandate is to improve the quality and relevance of evidence available to help patients, caregivers, clinicians, and other stakeholders make informed health decisions. Specifically, PCORI funds comparative clinical effectiveness research (CER), as well as work that will improve the methods used to conduct such studies. For example, PCORI currently funds a project involving the adequacy of surveillance following breast cancer treatment.

Future Programs

MACRA, MIPS, and APMs

On April 16, 2015, President Obama signed into law the Medicare Access and Children's Health Insurance Program Reauthorization Act (MACRA). The enactment of MACRA culminated a 15-year effort to repeal the Medicare sustainable growth rate (SGR), which calculated payment cuts for physicians. MACRA establishes an alternative set of predictable annual baseline payment updates incorporating two major provisions under the overarching name of the Quality Payment Program (QPP): the Merit-based Incentive Payment System (MIPS) and incentive payments for participation in certain Alternative Payment Models (APMs). Full implementation occurs in 2019 with data collection beginning in 2017.

The MIPS statute integrates and aligns the PQRS, VBM, and EHR Incentive Program into a single performance program. MIPS will be a robust quality and performance improvement program that establishes a composite score for each physician in four domains: quality, resource utilization, meaningful use, and clinical practice improvement activities. Each of these domains will be assigned a percentage of the total composite score, which will change over time. Physicians will then be judged based upon this composite score. Physicians scoring in the lowest quartile will automatically be adjusted down to the maximum penalty for the performance year. Physicians scoring in the highest quartile are eligible for a potential positive payment adjustment up to the maximum gain. As mentioned earlier, performance periods are likely to predate payment periods by 2 years.

The quality components of MIPS will be based on the quality measures currently used in the quality performance programs with additional measures solicited by the HHS Secretary from professional organizations and others in the healthcare community. Each year, the HHS Secretary will publish a list of quality measures to be used in the forthcoming MIPS performance period through the normal rulemaking process. Physicians will select which measures on the final list to report and be assessed on them. MIPS has a priority to utilize outcome measures and measures that are relevant for specialty providers. Among these, patient reported outcome measures (PROMs) are of the utmost importance. However, at present PROM development is still in its early stages, particularly as it relates to physician reimbursement.

The MACRA legislation also aims to stimulate high value care by promoting and incentivizing participation in APMs. Current fee-for-service (FFS) payment systems prevent the implementation of changes in care delivery needed to maximize quality. For instance, practices lose revenue if surgeons perform fewer procedures or lower-cost procedures. APMs support the delivery of higher quality care for patients at lower costs for purchasers in ways that are financially feasible for physician practices. There are several different types of APMs, some of which evolved in the private sector, others which were established by the ACA. The ACA created the Center for Medicare and Medicaid Innovation (CMMI) to develop and test value-based alternative payment methods. Examples of current APMs include the Medicare Shared Savings Program (MSSP) for Accountable Care Organizations (ACOs), the patient-centered medical home (PCMH) model, and the Bundled Payments for Care Improvement (BCPI) initiative.

Under a bundled, or capitated, payment arrangement, payers compensate physicians with a single payment for an episode of care, which is defined as a set of services delivered to a patient over a specific time period. This model aims to incentivize providers to improve care coordination, limit costly and unnecessary services, and reduce variations in care not tied to patient care quality and outcomes. By providing one single payment for various providers, bundled payments seek to promote a team-based approach to care. Though bundled payments differ based on the patients' illnesses and conditions, and tend to reflect the average costs of the treatments involved in an episode of care, they do not typically vary with the explicit number or mix of services provided to any individual patient. For example, Geisinger Health Plan established ProvenCare, a bundled payment program that pays one fee for the surgical episode of care, including pre- and postoperative services for coronary bypass, hip replacement, cataract surgery, and bariatric surgery. In most bundled payment models, participating providers share in savings if their actual expenditures are below the bundled payment amount.

Public Reporting

Multi-stakeholder, consensus-based quality measurement is central to the delivery of safe, accessible, patient-centered, and affordable care. Surgeons recognize that the clinical responsibility entrusted to them is based on accountability to the patient. The scope of that accountability includes commitments to appropriate and effective therapy, patient safety, and optimal clinical outcomes. While these commitments are implied in the social contract with the patient, both public and private agencies publically report on these aspects of care at the institutional and now often surgeon level. In fact, public reporting is mandated by federal legislation. While the intents are to increase transparency in healthcare, to assist patients in making informed decisions about their healthcare choices, and to encourage providers to identify opportunities for improvement, many current reports are not reliably consistent or accurate. Herein we describe how public reporting might be appropriately used to support surgical quality improvement efforts and how it might be refined to achieve intended goals.

Current Issues in Public Reporting

Data Source

All healthcare data collection and reporting modalities suffer from inherent limitations. For instance, the claims data that commercial payers and CMS currently use are designed primarily for billing and payment purposes, so-called "administrative data", and are not specifically tailored for quality measurement. They are accessible in large numbers, and are thus relatively inexpensive to analyze. They often allow for easy identification of sociodemographic patterns of healthcare access. However, administrative data do not address the nuances of comorbidities, disease severity, conditions present on admission, postoperative complications, and patient-reported outcomes. Therefore, these claims data are ineffective for tracking many relevant clinical processes and outcomes. In fact, CMS has recognized the limitations of claims-based data, acknowledging that it has been created for billing purposes and not for quality reporting.

Documentation and coding gaps are major drawbacks for utilizing administrative data. Hospitals' medical records staffs, who are not directly involved in patient care, are limited by the information documented in the medical record. Documentation by the surgeon is therefore of the utmost importance as any inappropriate or omitted data are carried over to benchmarking reports utilizing these data. Furthermore, ambiguity in documentation can lead to misinterpretation by medical records staff, thereby adding bias or outright error. Hospital coding also aggregates specific diagnosis codes into diagnosis-related groups (DRGs) that define reimbursement rather than reflect an accurate sequence of clinical events representative of the clinical care delivered.

Whereas feedback from outcomes data to physicians and hospitals can be a powerful tool in quality improvement, an overreliance on claims data is problematic. Indeed, the crucial ability to risk-adjust at the individual patient level to account for differences in patient case-mix and other factors affecting procedural risk remains limited despite the many algorithms that attempt to compensate for these deficiencies. Ideally, surgical care should be assessed with clinical data, such as those obtained by the ACS National Surgical Quality Improvement Project (NSQIP), using outcomes measures specifically designed for surgical quality improvement that are clinically relevant and risk-adjusted (Cohen et al. 2013). These data may then be combined with episode-based and long-term resource use data that assess cost as a way to measure and improve value. However, clinical data can be expensive and often difficult to obtain due to the inherent variation in how hospitals and physicians collect and document data.

A recent pilot project with AHRQ and the Minnesota Hospital Association found that the use of hybrid data allowed for more accurate comparisons of risk-adjusted outcomes across Minnesota hospitals (Pine et al. 2012). In the future, automatic abstraction from EHRs might substantially improve the cost, quality and access to relevant, timely clinical information. Further research is needed to evaluate the potential of hybrid data and automatic abstraction.

Attribution

The complexity of many surgical treatments, particularly in oncology, requires a team of physicians with complementary skills to achieve optimal patient outcomes. Unfortunately, no standardized methodology is available to appropriately distinguish between individual providers from a team who participate in the patient episodes of care, and to appropriately assign accountability for that care. Current methodologies can rely on identifying the physician who provided the majority of the patient's care as defined by the number of specific services or charges, or simply identify the admitting, discharging, or proceduralist physician. This, in the context of aggregated administrative data, prevents the attribution of adverse events to specific providers. For instance, the surgeon may unintentionally be attributed elements of a patient's care that the he or she may have little control over, such as imaging and other tests. Appropriate attribution, either to individual providers or to a group of multiple providers, can dramatically affect the accuracy of public reports.

Improving Public Reporting

Variability

Although public reports are widely available, the content, design, and availability of reports may hinder their successful utilization to drive improvement. Few reports are well-tailored to patients' needs (Sinaiko et al. 2012). Each report represents multiple decisions about what type of information to include, underlying differences in methodology, and presentation style. Certainly, two organizations could each use the same underlying data, but produce two reports presenting different results (Hwang et al. 2014; Leonardi et al. 2007). For example, Rothberg et al. compared the hospital ratings of five popular websites: CMS's *Hospital Compare*, Health Grades, the Leapfrog Group, US News and World Report, and Massachusetts Healthcare Quality and Cost (Rothberg et al. 2008). The authors found no consistency in the level of agreement of hospital rankings between the websites and concluded that a lack of uniformity in reporting might actually be contrary to the well-intended efforts of public reporting.

Transparency and Inclusion

To improve the accuracy of published measurements, public reports should make available their methodology both to the patients and to the providers they intend to describe (Damberg et al. 2014). Misclassification of the quality performance of surgeons can be mitigated through the use of rigorous statistical analysis, particularly for risk adjustment. The data source, selected performance measures, and period of data collection should also be published. It is important to clearly define the "numerator" and the "denominator" of the quality measures being applied. For example, a quality measure in melanoma care proposed by the Commission on Cancer (CoC) penalizes sentinel lymph node biopsies performed on patients with thin melanomas. However, it is imperative to know whether concessions are made for patients who have thin melanomas with high-risk features. The point in time at which the outcome is measured should also be clearly described. This will provide the patient with a more accurate snapshot of the care being measured and help set expectations. For instance, 30-day outcomes are most appropriate when measuring immediate postoperative complications from an oncologic resection, while follow up on the order of years is most appropriate for measuring cancer-specific outcomes.

Surgeons are inherently well-suited to examine the validity of public reports. Having quality measures and public reports developed and reviewed by surgeons is imperative for validity. In fact, an appeals process might also be useful. In this way, inaccuracies that have the potential to affect a surgeon's reputation and practice can be addressed appropriately. Surgical societies, such as the ACS, can facilitate such exchanges to improve the quality of surgical care.

Risk Adjustment

There can be vast differences in the course of disease or response to care between groups of patients with the same diagnoses. The variations between patients are difficult to measure and have significant implications on surgical decision-making. These patient-attributable characteristics that increase the complexity of surgical care are difficult to accurately convey in public reporting. For instance, a patient who has previously undergone an abdominal operation is at increased risk for a more complicated subsequent abdominal operation. Disparities in access to surgical care, influenced by insurance coverage or location of patient residence, have also been shown to affect patient outcomes. Appropriate risk-adjustment methodologies can reduce unfair comparisons between surgeons based on the case-mix of patients.

Reliability

Statistical reliability represents the ability to detect the "signal" from the "noise" of a specific performance measure (Huffman et al. 2015). It quantifies the degree to which a calculated performance measure is based on actual differences in performance compared to measurement error. Case volume and event rate are important factors driving reliability, but so is the distribution of performance across providers. Hall et al. utilized the ACS NSQIP to study individual surgeon profiling paying attention to reliability of assessment (Hall et al. 2015). They demonstrated individual surgeons could be reliably differentiated when comparing their morbidity and surgical site infection outcomes, but less so for mortality because of the low event rate. For mortality to be a statistically reliable measure of individual surgeon performance, approximately 570 operative cases per surgeon would be required. Therefore, not all quality measures can be reliably measured and reported for all surgeons given the limitations of statistical methodology and operative volumes. Minimum case numbers or measures of reliability should be published to improve the validity of public reporting.

Influencing the Surgeon

Public reporting provides the opportunity for surgeons to reflect upon the quality of care they provide to their patients by comparing themselves with their peers to identify areas for potential improvement. Properly conducted, public reporting can lead to changes in quality due to changes in provider behavior rather than by biased selection of providers by patients (Totten et al. 2012). To effectively promulgate positive change, the information published by public reports need to be relevant, timely, complete, and accurate to carry validity and create trust. Furthermore, the emphasis should remain on improving the quality of care for our patients (Lamb et al. 2013). De-identification of surgeons in reports and a commitment to appropriately using performance reports for quality improvement are imperative to meeting the intended goals.

Surgeon Performance Reports

Physician Compare

CMS created the *Physician Compare* website on December 30, 2010 as mandated by the ACA (Centers for Medicare and Medicaid Services 2016). The goals aligned with those of public reporting: to provide information to help consumers make informed decisions and create clear incentives for physicians to perform well. Currently, Physician Compare makes public individual surgeon information regarding demographics, clinical training, hospital affiliation, American Board of Medical Specialties (ABMS) certification, and participation in any CMS quality programs, such as PQRS.

Quality measure data on 66 group practices participating in the PQRS Group Practice Reporting Option (GPRO) Incentive Program were initially reported in 2014. Group practices can have up to 14 quality measures on their profile page, as well as up to eight patient experience measures. Quality measures for individual providers began in late 2015 and will have full implementation by the end of 2016.

ProPublica's Surgeon Scorecard

ProPublica is an independent, non-profit public watchdog with the mission to expose abuses of public trust using investigative journalism. In July 2015, ProPublica published its online Surgeon Scorecard, which reports the performance of individual, identified surgeons for eight surgical procedures using Medicare data from 2009 to 2013 (Wei et al. 2015). They devised a novel composite measure incorporating death and readmissions within 30 days postoperatively and have marketed this as an "adjusted complication rate" for patients to interpret. However, substantial methodologic concerns have been raised (Friedberg et al. 2015). Key concerns include: statistical inaccuracies, inappropriate risk-adjustment, random misclassification of surgeon performance, failure to address hospital variation, and lack of external review by surgeons or other stakeholders prior to publication. There is concern that the reports will mislead and misinform patients.

Conclusions

Extensive efforts to improve surgical quality at the national level have been occurring at multiple levels in the form of regulations and public reporting. The need for improved quality in healthcare is well recognized and is reflected by numerous governmental agencies, such as AHRQ and PCORI, and private, non-profit organizations, such as the ACS, with the same mission to maximize the quality, safety, and access of healthcare services. Regulations at the surgeon level to improve quality are changing in the future with the passage of MACRA and the formation of the MIPS program. Understanding these regulatory changes will allow surgeons to maintain their leadership in the arena of quality improvement. Furthermore, the increasing emphasis on healthcare transparency through the public reporting of outcomes based on quality makes it imperative that all stakeholders be better educated on issues of reliability in order to minimize unintended and undesired consequences. Surgeons must embrace a culture of continuous measurement and improvement, and efforts need to be multidisciplinary collaborations involving all stakeholders.

Disclosures The authors have no financial disclosures or conflicts of interest to report related to this work.

References

American College of Surgeons. Overview of Medicare Quality Programs. 2016 [cited 2016 February 19]; Available from: https://www.facs.org/advocacy/quality/medicare-programs.

Centers for Medicare and Medicaid Services. 2016 PQRS Measures List. 2016 [cited 2016 February 29]; Available from: https://www.facs.org/~/media/files/advocacy/regulatory/pqrs_2016_measure_list.ashx.

Centers for Medicare and Medicaid Services. Physician Compare. 2016 [cited 2016 February 19]; Available from: https://www.medicare.gov/physiciancompare/.

Centers for Medicare and Medicaid Services. Regulations and Guidance. 2016 [cited 2016 February 19]; Available from: https://www.cms.gov/Regulations-and-Guidance/Regulations-and-Guidance.html.

Cohen ME, et al. Optimizing ACS NSQIP modeling for evaluation of surgical quality and risk: patient risk adjustment, procedure mix adjustment, shrinkage adjustment, and surgical focus. J Am Coll Surg. 2013;217(2):336–46. e1.

Damberg CL, Hyman D, France J. Do public reports of provider performance make their data and methods available and accessible? Med Care Res Rev. 2014;71(5 Suppl):81S–96.

Friedberg MW, et al. A Methodological Critique of the ProPublica Surgeon Scorecard. Santa Monica, CA: RAND Corporation, 2015. http://www.rand.org/pubs/perspectives/PE170.html.

Hall BL, et al. Profiling individual surgeon performance using information from a high-quality clinical registry: opportunities and limitations. J Am Coll Surg. 2015;221(5):901–13.

Healthcare Cost and Utilization Project (HCUP). Overview of the National (Nationwide) Inpatient Sample (NIS). 2015 [cited 2016 February 29]; Available from: https://www.hcup-us.ahrq.gov/nisoverview.jsp.

Huffman KM, et al. A comprehensive evaluation of statistical reliability in ACS NSQIP profiling models. Ann Surg. 2015;261(6):1108–13.

Hwang W, et al. Finding order in chaos: a review of hospital ratings. Am J Med Qual. 2014;31(2):147–55.

Lamb GC, et al. Publicly reported quality-of-care measures influenced Wisconsin physician groups to improve performance. Health Aff (Millwood). 2013;32(3):536–43.

Leonardi MJ, McGory ML, Ko CY. Publicly available hospital comparison web sites: determination of useful, valid, and appropriate information for comparing surgical quality. Arch Surg. 2007;142(9):863–8; discussion 868–9.

Pine M, et al. Harnessing the power of enhanced data for healthcare quality improvement: lessons from a Minnesota Hospital Association Pilot Project. J Healthc Manag. 2012;57(6):406–18; discussion 419–20.

Rothberg MB, et al. Choosing the best hospital: the limitations of public quality reporting. Health Aff (Millwood). 2008;27(6):1680–7.

Sinaiko AD, Eastman D, Rosenthal MB. How report cards on physicians, physician groups, and hospitals can have greater impact on consumer choices. Health Aff (Millwood). 2012;31(3):602–11.

Totten AM, et al. Closing the quality gap: revisiting the state of the science (vol. 5: public reporting as a quality improvement strategy). Evid Rep Technol Assess (Full Rep). 2012;(208.5):1–645.

U.S. Department of Health and Human Services. 2011 Report to Congress: National Strategy for Quality Improvement in Health Care. 2011; Available from: http://www.ahrq.gov/workingfor-quality/reports/annual-reports/nqs2011annlrpt.htm#s4next.

Wei S, Pierce O, Allen M. Surgeon Scorecard. 2015 [cited 2016 February 19]; Available from: https://projects.propublica.org/surgeons/.

Chapter 13
The Public Perception of Quality Improvement in Surgery

James Taylor, Tim Xu, and Martin A. Makary

Abstract Variation in the quality of health care patients receive is endemic, and medical errors (at both the provider and system levels) now rank as the third leading cause of death in the U.S. An analysis of surgeons performing colectomy procedures over a two-year period in Maryland showed that risk-adjusted complication rates varied between zero and ten times the average complication rate. Given these hazards, the public is eager to receive information to help them navigate the system to find reliable, state-of-the art surgical care.

Variation in the quality of health care patients receive is endemic, and medical errors (at both the provider and system levels) now rank as the third leading cause of death in the U.S. (Makary and Daniel 2016). An analysis of surgeons performing colectomy procedures over a two-year period in Maryland showed that risk-adjusted complication rates varied between zero and ten times the average complication rate (Xu et al. 2016). Given these hazards, the public is eager to receive information to help them navigate the system to find reliable, state-of-the art surgical care.

Public interest in surgical quality has grown vastly over the past decade. Until recently, patients had almost no worthwhile data beyond claims of individual centers or unadjusted cardiac surgery mortality data in certain states. But today, new apps are flushing through big data in an attempt to steer patients to high-quality, low-cost medical care. These resources are sending the general population more information than at any other point in history. The question we now face is: 'Are the data reliable, fair, and measuring the right things?'

J. Taylor, MBBChir, MPH
General Surgery Resident, Department of Surgery, Johns Hopkins University School of Medicine, Baltimore, MD, USA

T. Xu, MPP
Department of Surgery, Johns Hopkins University School of Medicine, Baltimore, MD, USA

M.A. Makary, MD, MPH (✉)
Johns Hopkins University School of Medicine, Health Policy & Management, Johns Hopkins Bloomberg School of Public Health, Baltimore, MD, USA
e-mail: mmakary1@jhmi.edu

© Springer International Publishing Switzerland 2017
R.R. Kelz, S.L. Wong (eds.), *Surgical Quality Improvement*,
Success in Academic Surgery, DOI 10.1007/978-3-319-23356-7_13

How this information is accrued, disseminated and interpreted ranges from sloppy to sophisticated, and the literature surrounding the subject remains in its infancy. This chapter will explore the trend towards public engagement in data and the relative merits and limitations, as well as future strategies to improve the transparency of surgical quality.

Does the Public Have a Right to Know?

At the crux of the public reporting discussion is the fundamental question: 'Does the public have a right to know about the quality of their community hospital?' Now that risk-adjusted complication rates and patterns of outlier practice patterns exist in taxpayer-funded datasets, notably those from the Centers for Medicaid and Medicare Services (CMS), does the public have a right to see it? The alternatives provide little to no information. Physicians who refer patients to surgeons rarely have access to concrete outcomes data. The medical malpractice system is a flawed screening mechanism for quality because it cannot capture a physician with a 50 % rate of complications since each patient harmed experiences the complication as a waived right as a part of informed consent. The pattern of complications is invisible to a patient and the malpractice system.

While the vast majority of surgeons care deeply about their patients and practice sound medicine, there are outliers who disproportionately harm a lot of patients. Should these outliers be reported, now that they can be identified with data, and do we as surgeons have a moral obligation to do something about these outliers? It has been our position that we do have an obligation as a profession to help outliers, beginning with sharing their outlier results with them directly—in a confidential, non-punitive, peer-to-peer fashion.

Improving Wisely

The national Robert Wood Johnson Foundation—SAGES—Johns Hopkins project shares data reports with surgeons on their individual performance as a courtesy to them ahead of what is anticipated to be public reporting of the same data by third parties. This friendly data sharing allows surgeons to see how they would look benchmarked to others and offers them tele-mentoring, coaching and resources available through SAGES. The project, called 'Improving Wisely', is based on early successes seen with The Society of Vascular Surgery and the American College of Mohs Surgeons members "auto-correcting" their performance with data-sharing alone. Public reporting of quality data is in strong demand by payers and patients. It is generally recognized that 10 years from now, nearly all quality data will be made public. Already Medicare has announced plans to disclose data with physician NPI numbers and they have launched a new website, physiciancompare.hhs.gov, which they hope to populate with meaningful specialty association-endorsed metrics in the future. The Improving Wisely initiative seeks to address outlier practice patterns around best practices in an "in-house" fashion ahead of a future trend toward public reporting.

Hospital and Physician Ratings

One of the highest profile public reporting resources is the hospital and specialty-specific rankings released on a yearly basis by US News and World Reporting (USNWR). These rankings, which are generated by a scoring system derived from a physician survey, mortality rate and observable hospital characteristics, are available in the USNWR magazine and online, so most people can gain access to them if they desire. Research has shown that hospitals use these rankings as an advertising aid and that rankings can have a significant impact on patient decision making, with higher rankings equating to higher patient influx and improved outcomes (Pope 2009; Sinaiko et al. 2012; Chen et al. 1999). Despite these positive correlations identified between hospital ranking and outcomes, other studies have discovered that there may in fact be no correlation at all. For example, Mulvey and colleagues showed that there was no association between a hospital's USNWR ranking and patient readmissions (Mulvey et al. 2009). Another conundrum identified in various studies is that there exists vast discrepancies between other highly regarded and widely accessed rating systems, such as the CMS Hospital Compare, HealthGrades, the Leapfrog Group and Consumer Reports (Halasyamani and Davis 2007; Osborne et al. 2011; Osborne et al. 2010; Austin et al. 2015). One potential resulting effect is that a hospital may be puzzlingly considered both a "high" and "low" performer, depending upon which rating system is referenced (Rothberg et al. 2008). The variation between rating systems has been closely studied and attributed to the use of different measures and foci, however great confusion can be created for patients as a result of a lack of methodological transparency (Austin et al. 2015). The field of public reporting struggles with finding meaningful metrics. As metrics of patient-centered quality mature over time, these websites will be better informed with more meaningful information.

The public's perception of surgical quality is further influenced by a number of online tools that allow for individual physicians or hospitals to be directly compared. Drawing from the data collected by CMS, patients are able to search by specialty or location and directly observe comparisons in a variety of areas (Medicare. Medicare.gov Physician Compare 2016). The aim, according to the Medicare website, is to aid users in making an informed decision about their medical care, however there are limitations, including the fact that only Medicare patient data is included in the comparisons of physicians. The CMS data has been further dissected by ProPublica, an independent, non-profit newsroom that claim to produce investigative journalism in the public interest. They created the "Surgeon Scorecard", which calculated risk-adjusted complication rates for surgeons performing very-low risk procedures in Medicare (Wei et al. 2015). To date, information is available on nearly 17,000 surgeons who performed the eight elective low-risk procedures. While the vast majority of surgeons in the dataset perform well, the analysis found that complication rates of an individual practitioner can be highly variable, even within hospitals that have good ratings and outcomes. The analysis responds to growing frustration by the public that health care has not disclosed outcomes.

Allowing patients to see the complication rate of their surgeon prior to deciding to go under the knife has been met with mixed reviews, with opinions divided as to whether the public truly benefit from seeing individualized data. Popular arguments in favor of ProPublica's work include providing a "tool to gather information about quality" upon which patients will be able to "make an informed choice about surgery," and that the public are able to see that "there is significant variation in the quality and safety outcomes of individual surgeons" (ProPublica. What Experts Are Saying About Surgeon Scorecard 2015). Those against releasing the data applied a high level of scrutiny to the methodology—a level of scrutiny that would crush most surgical studies published in the *New England Journal of Medicine* and *JAMA*, including those published by the critics themselves (ProPublica 2015; Freidberg et al. 2014; Jaffe et al. 2016; Auffenberg et al. 2016). For example, all scholars of safety have celebrated the reductions in hospital all-cause readmission rates with public reporting of hospital readmission rates, yet the same critics dismiss the notion that these readmission rates are meaningful at the provider level, even when the readmission are only counted if they are surgical complication-related and measured only for low-risk procedures. While no data analysis is perfect, the surgeon-led push back of the ProPublica data transparency initiative was territorial rather than scientific. Fortunately, surgeons are closely involved in revising the methodology so that version 2.0 will be better refined and conducted with a sense of surgeon participation (Allen and Pierce 2015). ProPublica has the potential to greatly impact a patient's decision regarding surgeon selection, but just how significant this impact is remains to be seen while the web tool is still in its early stages. Already payers and third party patient navigation companies are using the data.

Official rankings, ratings and statistically calculated tools are not the only place online that patients are turning to discover information about surgical quality. While the majority of the population may not be too familiar with CMS or ProPublica, physician-rating websites are becoming increasingly popular. These websites enable physicians to be compared to others, with ratings and comments left by patients and other parties. Physicians can be reviewed in the same manner that one might review a restaurant, with results presented in easy to comprehend ways that one might expect when browsing for a vacation on Trip Advisor. As social media continues to evolve and increase in popularity, even websites like Yelp and Facebook are being are being utilized to leave performance feedback and register satisfaction.

Some controversy exists surrounding the use of social media and physician-rating websites, as patients frequently leave comments related to the quality of parking at a hospital and the punctuality and bedside manner of a physician far more frequently than they do 'surgical quality' (Gao et al. 2012). Lagu and colleagues suggest that patients are offered a novel way to provide feedback and obtain information about individual performance (Lagu et al. 2010), with much support coming from the British Nation Health Service (Bacon 2009). Groups within the US have been hesitant to back such websites, with fear that reviews will be too negative (Dolan 2008) or that too many reviews will be falsified or posted by health care providers themselves (Solomon 2007). A lack of regulation and an inability for physicians to reply to feedback due to potential HIPAA violations raises additional concern about the legitimacy and effectiveness of these sites.

We believe that patient satisfaction (i.e. consumer ratings) have a place in health care quality but that it should not be regarded as a comprehensive metric of surgical quality (Gao et al. 2012). For example, appropriateness of care - one of the most important aspects of quality - is not captured in the metric. In fact, a patient can have an unnecessary operation and be joyfully satisfied with it. Similarly, pediatricians that inappropriately dispense antibiotics for viral upper respiratory infections can have higher patient satisfaction scores then those who are judicious and practice sound medicine.

The increasing popularity of rating websites and social media has prompted a plethora of research into the topic. One of the fundamental questions that has been asked is: "does patient satisfaction equate to quality process and outcomes?" and no clear answer appears to be evident. Lyu et al examined at how patient satisfaction correlated with surgical process measures, including prophylaxis, hair removal, Foley catheter removal, deep vein thrombosis prophylaxis, and hospital safety (Lyu et al. 2013). They discovered that patient satisfaction was independent of hospital compliance with surgical processes of quality care and with overall hospital employee safety culture. Conversely, a study looking at Facebook ratings and 30-day readmission rates found that the average ratings were higher for those hospitals with lower readmissions, with statistically significant differences between different star ratings (Glover et al. 2015). What is notable is that different metrics are utilized between studies, which makes direct comparison of research and formation of a definitive opinion difficult regarding the validity of rating websites that are highly influenced by patient satisfaction (Segal et al. 2012). An additional monkey wrench was thrown into the works when Manary and his co-authors further dissected the correlation between patient satisfaction and quality (Manary et al. 2013). They identified three major concerns regarding patient-reported measures that undermined the importance of satisfaction. Firstly, they noted that patients lack formal medical training and therefore are not in a position to appropriately assess surgical quality. Secondly, they suggest that satisfaction could be confounded by factors that are not directly associated with the quality of processes, such as their overall health status. A final concern is that patient satisfaction may be a reflection of whether patients received their *a priori* wishes, including whether or not they received a specific treatment or medication.

Other sources exist for patients to discover information relating to surgical quality, although the quality of these sources are themselves highly debatable. Numerous magazines and periodicals publish data on the 'top surgeons' in a region, though often not specifying how or why those surgeons are selected. Physicians may also give advice to patients about who they should choose to perform certain procedures. Though some may see this as an ideal, insiders-view, there may be other factors that influence referrals including financial or personal biases. Finally, surgeons or hospitals often attempt to lure patients with advertisements and billboards, utilizing selective reporting of quality data in an attempt to persuade the public.

The Future of Surgical Quality

Less than 1 % of surgical outcomes in the U.S. are captured today (Makary 2015). As metrics mature and the capture rate of patient outcomes increases in surgery, public reporting will become more meaningful. As surgeons, we need to ensure that any metric being applied privately or publically is fair. Risk-adjustment needs to be sound and consider the potential for physicians to game the system.

Hospital-specific and surgeon-specific data are expanding as patients and the public demand greater transparency of surgical quality (Makary 2012). The future of surgical quality reporting and the public's perception of that information are poised for change, with developments in technology and increasing access to quality-related statistics. One such avenue of development exists in the form of video technology, with some investigators having already demonstrated the potential of using video to improve safety practices within an OR (Overdyk et al. 2015). Video has been proposed as a tool to take quality to the next level and address endemic variation in surgical quality (Makary 2013). Video technology has also been used by surgeons to obtain feedback about their practice and skills from experts in that particular field (Hu et al. 2012), and Birkmeyer et al. have looked at peer-rated video footage to describe variation in surgeon technical skill and its association with complication, readmission and mortality rates (Birkmeyer et al. 2013). Issues of confidentiality and malpractice exposure have been addressed and need to be ever present when implementing video-recording in the practice of medicine (Joo et al. 2016). Despite these fears, video has the potential to increase transparency, accountability and the overall quality of surgical care when used properly. In the past video recording was not feasible, but given advances in data storage and the ease of recording video based procedures today, it represents a tremendous opportunity.

One of the major barriers that stand in the way of increased transparency and advancements in surgical quality are surgeons themselves. Surgeons have been found to be in favor of public reporting on an aggregate level, but are far less supportive of individual-surgeon-level data. There is concern about the method and interpretation of reported statistics, particularly related to patient understanding and the availability of validated outcome metrics that appropriately adjust for case-specific risk (Sherman et al. 2013). The consequences of public reporting also result in surgeon apprehension, with the fear that surgeons may choose to only operate on healthier, low-risk patients to improve their outcome data.

People travel from all across the country to undergo select procedures at hospitals based upon the hospital or surgeon reputation and rating, or thanks to recommendations from friends, colleagues or other medical providers. It is a very difficult task to objectively evaluate the surgical quality of a particular surgeon or institution, especially with so many different sources of information and with great variation amongst the metrics used to represent quality. Until we have more mature metrics and until patient outcomes are captured at a higher rate, public perception can be greatly influenced by popular media, particularly with the evolution of rating websites. Just how closely correlated a 5-star rating on Yelp or Facebook relates to surgical quality is a topic of great contention and debate (Rajaram et al. 2015). Moreover, as hospitals increasingly seek to distinguish themselves from the competition, inaccurate or false advertising about measures of quality may lead to patients receiving sub-optimal care. For all these reasons, public perception of quality depends on surgeons and policymakers coming together to develop strong metrics of surgical quality.

Surgical care is a service provided by not only an individual surgeon, but rather a team that includes everyone from the receptionist that patients encounter in clinic to the nursing teams that provide day-to-day postoperative care. Measuring the quality of the care that the team renders remains a scientific field in evolution.

References

Allen M, Pierce O. MAKING THE CUT. Why choosing the right surgeon matters even more than you know 2015 [cited 2016 February 21st]. Available from: https://www.propublica.org/article/surgery-risks-patient-safety-surgeon-matters.

Auffenberg GB, Ghani KR, Ye Z, Dhir A, Gao Y, Stork B, et al. Comparing publicly reported surgical outcomes with quality measures from a statewide improvement collaborative. JAMA Surg. 2016;151(7):680–2.

Austin JM, Jha AK, Romano PS, Singer SJ, Vogus TJ, Wachter RM, et al. National hospital ratings systems share few common scores and may generate confusion instead of clarity. Health Aff (Millwood). 2015;34(3):423–30.

Bacon N. Will doctor rating sites improve standards of care? Yes. BMJ. 2009;338:b1030.

Birkmeyer JD, Finks JF, O'Reilly A, Oerline M, Carlin AM, Nunn AR, et al. Surgical skill and complication rates after bariatric surgery. N Engl J Med. 2013;369(15):1434–42.

Chen J, Radford MJ, Wang Y, Marciniak TA, Krumholz HM. Do "America's Best Hospitals" perform better for acute myocardial infarction? N Engl J Med. 1999;340(4):286–92.

Dolan P. Patients rarely use online ratings to pick physicians 2008 [cited 2016 February 22nd]. Available from: http://www.ama-assn.org/amednews/2008/06/23/bil10623.htm.

Freidberg MW, Pronovost PJ, Shahian DM, Safran DG, Bilimoria KY, Elliott MN, et al. A methodological critique of the ProPublica surgeon scorecard: RAND; 2014 [cited 2016 March 22nd]. Available from: http://www.rand.org/pubs/perspectives/PE170.html.

Gao GG, McCullough JS, Agarwal R, Jha AK. A changing landscape of physician quality reporting: analysis of patients' online ratings of their physicians over a 5-year period. J Med Internet Res. 2012;14(1), e38.

Glover M, Khalilzadeh O, Choy G, Prabhakar AM, Pandharipande PV, Gazelle GS. Hospital evaluations by social media: a comparative analysis of facebook ratings among performance outliers. J Gen Intern Med. 2015;30(10):1440–6.

Halasyamani LK, Davis MM. Conflicting measures of hospital quality: ratings from "Hospital Compare" versus "Best Hospitals". J Hosp Med. 2007;2(3):128–34.

Hu YY, Peyre SE, Arriaga AF, Osteen RT, Corso KA, Weiser TG, et al. Postgame analysis: using video-based coaching for continuous professional development. J Am Coll Surg. 2012;214(1):115–24.

Jaffe TA, Hasday SJ, Dimick JB. Power outage-inadequate surgeon performance measures leave patients in the dark. JAMA Surg. 2016;151(7):599–600.

Joo S, Xu T, Makary MA. Video transparency: a powerful tool for patient safety and quality improvement. BMJ Qual Saf. 2016: 2016 Jan 28. pii: bmjqs-2015-005058. doi: 10.1136/bmjqs-2015-005058. [Epub ahead of print].

Lagu T, Hannon NS, Rothberg MB, Lindenauer PK. Patients' evaluations of health care providers in the era of social networking: an analysis of physician-rating websites. J Gen Intern Med. 2010;25(9):942–6.

Lyu H, Wick EC, Housman M, Freischlag JA, Makary MA. Patient satisfaction as a possible indicator of quality surgical care. JAMA Surg. 2013;148(4):362–7.

Makary MA. Unaccountable. New York: Bloomsbury Press; 2012.

Makary MA. The power of video recording: taking quality to the next level. JAMA. 2013;309(15):1591–2.

Makary MA. Why our health care system is broken 2015 [cited 2016 March 22nd]. Available from: http://www.cnn.com/2015/12/22/opinions/makary-health-care-system/.

Makary MA, Daniel M. Medical error: the third leading cause of death in the U.S. BMJ. 2016;353:i2139.

Manary MP, Boulding W, Staelin R, Glickman SW. The patient experience and health outcomes. N Engl J Med. 2013;368(3):201–3.

Medicare. Medicare.gov Physician Compare 2016 [cited 2016 February 20th]. Available from: https://www.medicare.gov/PhysicianCompare/search.html.

Mulvey GK, Wang Y, Lin Z, Wang OJ, Chen J, Keenan PS, et al. Mortality and readmission for patients with heart failure among U.S. News & World Report's top heart hospitals. Circ Cardiovasc Qual Outcomes. 2009;2(6):558–65.

Osborne NH, Nicholas LH, Ghaferi AA, Upchurch Jr GR, Dimick JB. Do popular media and internet-based hospital quality ratings identify hospitals with better cardiovascular surgery outcomes? J Am Coll Surg. 2010;210(1):87–92.

Osborne NH, Ghaferi AA, Nicholas LH, Dimick JB, Mph M. Evaluating popular media and internet-based hospital quality ratings for cancer surgery. Arch Surg. 2011;146(5):600–4.

Overdyk FJ, Dowling O, Newman S, Glatt D, Chester M, Armellino D, et al. Remote video auditing with real-time feedback in an academic surgical suite improves safety and efficiency metrics: a cluster randomised study. BMJ Qual Saf. 2015.

Pope DG. Reacting to rankings: evidence from "America's Best Hospitals". J Health Econ. 2009;28(6):1154–65.

ProPublica. What Experts Are Saying About Surgeon Scorecard 2015 [cited 2016 February 21st]. Available from: https://www.propublica.org/article/surgeon-level-risk-quotes.

Rajaram R, Chung JW, Kinnier CV, Barnard C, Mohanty S, Pavey ES, et al. Hospital characteristics associated with penalties in the centers for Medicare & Medicaid services hospital-acquired condition reduction program. JAMA. 2015;314(4):375–83.

Rothberg MB, Morsi E, Benjamin EM, Pekow PS, Lindenauer PK. Choosing the best hospital: the limitations of public quality reporting. Health Aff (Millwood). 2008;27(6):1680–7.

Segal J, Sacopulos M, Sheets V, Thurston I, Brooks K, Puccia R. Online doctor reviews: do they track surgeon volume, a proxy for quality of care? J Med Internet Res. 2012;14(2), e50.

Sherman KL, Gordon EJ, Mahvi DM, Chung J, Bentrem DJ, Holl JL, et al. Surgeons' perceptions of public reporting of hospital and individual surgeon quality. Med Care. 2013;51(12):1069–75.

Sinaiko AD, Eastman D, Rosenthal MB. How report cards on physicians, physician groups, and hospitals can have greater impact on consumer choices. Health Aff (Millwood). 2012;31(3):602–11.

Solomon S. Doc's RateMDs battle turns ugly. National Review of Medicine. 2007 [cited 2016 February 22nd]. Available from: http://www.nationalreviewofmedicine.com/issue/2007/05_15/4_patients_practice09_9.html.

Wei S, Pierce O, Allen M. Surgeon Scorecard 2015 [cited 2016 February 20th]. Available from: https://projects.propublica.org/surgeons/.

Xu T, Makary MA, Kazzi EA, Zhou M, Pawlik TM, Hutfless SM. Surgeon-level variation in postoperative complications. J Gastrointest Surg. 2016;20(7):1393–9.

Index

© Springer International Publishing Switzerland 2017
R.R. Kelz, S.L. Wong (eds.), *Surgical Quality Improvement*,
Success in Academic Surgery, DOI 10.1007/978-3-319-23356-7

Printed in the United States
By Bookmasters